IMAGES
of America

MERCY FLIGHTS

ON THE COVER: Mercy Flights founder George Milligan is shown planning routes with the first group of volunteer pilots (from left to right): Bill Childers, Eugene Kooser, Dick Nyoff, Lee Flink, Harvey Brandau, Milligan, Jack Edmonds, Cecil Davis, and Fred Edens. As enthusiastic community pilots with extensive World War II flying experience, they were able to log valuable flying time while also saving lives. (Courtesy of Mercy Flights and the Southern Oregon Historical Society.)

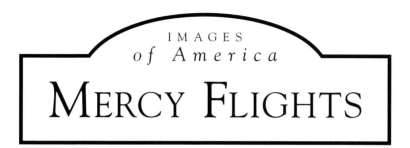

IMAGES
of America
MERCY FLIGHTS

Ruth Ballweg, Michael E. Burrill Sr.,
Michael E. Burrill Jr., and Pirkko Terao

ARCADIA
PUBLISHING

Published by Arcadia Publishing
Charleston, South Carolina

Printed in the United States of America

Library of Congress Control Number: 2017932521

For all general information, please contact Arcadia Publishing:
Telephone 843-853-2070
Fax 843-853-0044
E-mail sales@arcadiapublishing.com
For customer service and orders:
Toll-Free 1-888-313-2665

Visit us on the Internet at www.arcadiapublishing.com

*This book is dedicated to the patients, community volunteers,
board members, pilots, nurses, paramedics, and staff
members who personify the mission of Mercy Flights.*

Contents

Acknowledgments

This book would not have been possible without the support and guidance of Helene Milligan, widow of George Milligan. Additional credit must also be given to Jack Wheeler, who served as Mercy Flights' unofficial historian over the years and provided unlimited access to the entire collection, and Diane Coash, Mercy Flights' office manager, who helped provide names to accompany pictures and memories.

Several organizations and individuals helped in our research and provided images as noted. These include the Southern Oregon Historical Society; the Museum of Flight; the *Medford Mail Tribune*; Oregon Health & Science University Historical Collections & Archives; Providence Archives; Timberland Helicopters, Inc.; Marie Garsjo; Geoff Collins; Doug Stewart; Amy Hall; and Tim James.

We would also like to thank Hydrogen Advertising, based in Seattle, and their senior digital designer, Brian McCartney, for providing the tools and training needed to prepare all of the images reproduced on these pages.

Unless otherwise noted, all images used in this book come from the Mercy Flights collection.

INTRODUCTION

Mercy Flights, based in Medford, Oregon, and incorporated in 1949, was created by founder George Milligan to respond to the urgent needs of critically ill or injured residents of coastal Southern Oregon, Northern California, and Oregon who needed speedy transportation to receive specialized medical care only available outside their geographically isolated area. The polio epidemic of 1949 drove home this point, making patients and their families aware of the six hours of travel on two-lane roads that stood between them and the nearest iron lung or specialty medical and surgical care.

Describing the situation in his book, *Their Eyes on the Skies,* aviation writer Martin Cole stated: "In the rugged, wooded wilderness around Medford, Oregon, only two forms of transportation have ever worked really well: mules and airplanes. Most of the mules are gone. The airplane remains as the combination of Santa Claus and Florence Nightingale for thousands of Southern Oregonians and Northern Californians who choose to live and work so far from civilization that a cry for help can easily go unheard."

In the late 1940s, the growing community of Medford had new residents—military veterans—who were eager to contribute to their community. George Milligan, a federal employee of the Civil Aeronautics Authority (CAA) (now the Federal Aviation Administration [FAA]) and a pilot himself, became aware of the desperate need for medical help in the region. According to *Their Eyes on the Skies,* "When he heard the frantic calls asking for doctors and ambulances over the shortwave radio, he felt utter helplessness. He was a pilot, thinking as an airman would. In each instance, on hearing distress calls, he spotted the origin of the call on the tower map. Then he translated the distance to the nearest hospital in terms of air time."

Although he had no intention of becoming a civic leader, Milligan spoke with Medford mayor Diamond Flynn and said, "What this community needs is a volunteer rescue operation. I'd be willing to volunteer as a pilot." Mayor Flynn immediately connected him with recently arrived *Medford Mail Tribune* editor Eric Allen as the first step in what would become a major community endeavor. Allen was originally skeptical. Similar air ambulance models had been developed elsewhere; however, they had all proven to be unsustainable. Milligan convinced Allen that Medford was a unique community where citizens could unite to do something special.

Milligan and Allen strategized to recruit community leaders for a hardworking, effective, and influential board of directors, with members including the mayor, lumber company owners, orchardists, a popular minister, Medford's only female lawyer, an undertaker, and representatives of the medical community. The board took on fundraising, interactions with political leaders, policy development, and the development of a legal infrastructure for the fledgling organization. Allen made sure that Mercy Flights received excellent local and regional press coverage of its growth and development. Over time, this coverage included stories of courageous rescues, fundraising air shows, governmental obstacles, the acquisition of new planes, and the utilization of technology to provide safer and more comfortable transport for patients and their families.

In an impressive example of community activism, a variety of Southern Oregon residents—from business leaders to schoolchildren—banded together to help start a not-for-profit medical transport service, and Mercy Flights became a reality. The first plane—a war surplus Cessna—was purchased with $3,000 in proceeds from community-wide fundraising, including $1,000 that schoolchildren collected in milk cartons.

After the plane was purchased, the remaining funds were used to acquire radios and medical equipment. Later, Mercy Flights' first hangar was built with lumber donated from community lumber companies and time donated by loggers and construction workers. Local women's clubs provided food for the volunteers in what became a highly publicized hangar-raising event.

As an experienced pilot himself (and a full-time employee of the FAA), Milligan was able to attract former military pilots who needed hours in the air to maintain their licenses. Milligan also became a role model and mentor for younger pilots willing to serve as copilots to gain valuable flying experience.

The next challenge was to provide sustainable funding for the service. Mercy Flights carried seven patients in its first year and thirteen in its second year—of these 20 patients, 10 could not afford to pay for the service. The number of patients transported by Mercy Flights doubled and tripled in the third and fourth year as the polio epidemic raged and increased accidents and emergencies in remote areas on the Oregon Coast demonstrated the need for Mercy Flights' services.

Milligan came up with a subscription plan for residents of the region that would provide free medical transport—if needed—for the cost of $2 per year per family. While this was originally viewed with suspicion as a possible "communist/socialist plot" during the McCarthy era (in the early 1950s), the annual subscriptions became popular and were offered as benefits by many employers, especially in hazardous industries such as logging and construction. Subscription drives, managed and staffed by volunteers, were held at sporting events, county fairs, and parades. In addition, the subscriptions were readily available in local businesses such as utility companies, grocery stores, and medical facilities. Other funding came from air shows sponsored by local service clubs that featured tours of Mercy Flights aircraft hosted by volunteer pilots and nurses.

It soon became apparent that Mercy Flights had underestimated the need for its services. The founders had initially envisioned providing just a few flights per month. However, as the World War II pilots painted small red crosses (visible in early Mercy Flights photographs) on their aircraft to keep a tally of successful missions, they soon realized that they would quickly cover the entire surface of their planes with these red crosses and abandoned the plan.

In expanding their fleet, Mercy Flights replaced older planes and added newer, more adaptable ones. Through a complicated negotiation and an act of Congress sponsored by Oregon's congressional delegation, Mercy Flights, in partnership with Rogue Valley Hospital, obtained two Twin Beechcraft C45s, the military version of the Beech 18, from the US Air Force surplus depot in Arizona. Mercy Flights sold its Stinson Reliant to pay for the conversion of the two planes to civilian status so they could provide safer service for night and reduced-visibility operations.

The original Beech aircraft were later replaced with two newer versions from US Air Force surplus that were equipped with the company's first deicing systems. Milligan reported, "Subsequent progressive upgrading of specialized aircraft models has culminated in a four plane fleet which Mercy Flights now operates. These are: a Twin Beech; an Aero Commander 680#, a Piper Cherokee Six (one 300-hp engine) and a Cessna 180 with an enlarged loading door. Each aircraft fits a different and special purpose."

Shown in every early photograph of Mercy Flights planes are the major structural modifications that were required in order for staff to move patients in and out of the aircraft. Until 1967, neither single- nor twin-engine planes were manufactured with doors sufficiently large enough to load full-size stretchers. Thus, for the first 18 years of its existence, Mercy Flights had to design—and gain FAA approval—for a larger modified loading door on each plane it placed in service.

While it is difficult to imagine now, there were no organized or governmental rescue agencies in the United States prior to the passage of federal and state Emergency Medical Services (EMS) legislation in the late 1970s and early 1980s. There were no paramedics and no 911 services.

Ambulances primarily existed to transport patients to and from hospitals. Rescues and evacuations were carried out as the need arose by bystanders and volunteers, the Civil Air Patrol, and Boy Scout Explorer Posts. It is not surprising that Mercy Flights stepped into this vacuum and was soon involved in dramatic rescues from small remote airstrips, searches for downed aircraft, and supporting communities impacted by natural disasters and other tragedies.

Along the way, Mercy Flights saved many lives and participated in daring rescues—including providing blood and medical supplies to Roseburg, Oregon, when it was rocked by a dynamite explosion in its city center. In very small communities, Mercy Flights' small and adaptable single-engine air ambulance planes could touch down in remote areas where the landing strips were small and unlit. During precarious night landings, community members gathered together to light the runways with car headlights.

Initially, volunteer pilots and nurses donated their time—often at inconvenient times and in potentially dangerous conditions—to assure the rapid and efficient transport of seriously ill and injured patients. As the service grew, paid and on-call staff replaced many of the volunteers. Continuity in leadership provided by Milligan, the board, a chief nurse, and medical advisors became key to Mercy Flights' success.

On September 20, 1971, despite 22 years of safe and courageous service, Mercy Flights was suddenly notified by the FAA of their intent to ground Mercy Flights because it did not conform to federal air taxi regulations. Starting on Wednesday, October 20, 1971, a two-day hearing was held in Medford with local attorney Otto Frohnmayer representing Mercy Flights.

Mercy Flights spokespersons contended that air taxi regulations were written with "no thought for the kind of lifesaving operations by Mercy Flights." Common rescue challenges, such as landing at night on unlit airstrips, landing on highways, or flying in extreme weather conditions were prohibited by air taxi regulations. Other objections included concerns about the ruinous possibility that Mercy Flights would lose its nonprofit status and tax exemptions and thus be forced out of existence.

Evidence presented during the hearing included an outpouring of support from the isolated Southern Oregon Coast, including personal testimony, affidavits, letters, petitions, and the endorsement of Mercy Flights by Gov. Tom McCall and Sen. Mark Hatfield. Nevertheless, according to *Their Eyes on the Skies*, FAA representatives "gave every indication they were out to ground Mercy Flights. . . . Finally, as feared, a tentative finding was issued: Mercy Flights must be grounded."

The governor, Oregon's two senators, and four congressmen immediately responded. Feeling the pressure, the FAA sent one of their medical experts to visit, inspect, investigate, and evaluate Mercy Flights. Fortunately, the doctor chose to expand his visit to not just include an inspection of Mercy Flights Medford facilities, he also requested flights to Oregon coastal communities, small remote airstrips, and medical facilities throughout the region. The inspector concluded that not only was Mercy Flights safe, but that it should also be considered a model for other developing air ambulance services. In June 1972, the FAA and Mercy Flights reached an agreement that would allow Mercy Flights to continue operations.

Subsequently, Mercy Flights became the nation's first not-for profit air ambulance company, paving the way for similar developments across the nation. Mercy Flights—and Milligan—worked tirelessly with senators and congressmen to craft the first federal air ambulance rules and regulations to support patient services and thereby increase health-care access in rural and remote communities. This new federal infrastructure opened the door for the creation of a wide range of medical transport services—the air ambulance movement—across the United States.

In a celebratory article about Mercy Flights, *Medford Mail Tribune* editor and Mercy Flights board member Eric Allen wrote, "Only in Medford, is there an ambulance service which is not in business to make money, which is completely independent, which exists only to service the sick and injured and which is operated by a few dedicated souls whose only reward is the feeling of satisfaction they get by knowing they are performing a vital and important service to their fellow human beings."

Sadly, Mercy Flights history includes two tragic crashes: one in 1985 and a second in 1989. In February 1985, founder George Milligan, Dr. Henry Boehnke (a beloved Medford pediatrician serving as copilot), paramedic Steve Trosin, and an elderly patient were killed in a crash near the Medford airport when they were returning from Gold Beach on the Oregon Coast. In August 1989, a Mercy Flights Beechcraft King-Air crashed while landing in Gold Beach during foggy weather. The crew included pilot Richard Mendolia, copilot Wally Nitowski, and flight nurse Diane Lefler. Intensive investigations by the FAA were controversial. Fortunately, an effective board of directors moved quickly and effectively to assure the continuity of Mercy Flights.

Though the original goal of Mercy Flights was to transport patients to larger medical centers in Portland and San Francisco, this trend was reversed as Medford's two small community hospitals—Sacred Heart Hospital and Medford Community Hospital—were rebuilt, expanded, and renamed as Providence Hospital and Rogue Valley Memorial Hospital, respectively, and became tertiary care centers utilizing every possible category of medical and surgical specialists and subspecialists. Physicians and surgeons could be more easily recruited into a small community if that community had a readily available air ambulance service.

Advances in medical technology and medical training programs developed in the US military or at NASA allowed Mercy Flights to better serve families and patients in the region. New electronic monitoring techniques and advanced drug-delivery systems made transport routine when it previously would have been impossible. Advanced training for nurses and the creation of emergency medical technician (EMT) and paramedic programs expanded the medical transport workforce. Mercy Flights became an early adopter of all of these innovations and hired some of the first flight nurses and paramedics as they became available.

Over time, Mercy Flights was able to develop additional focus on more complex medical transfers. New developments in aviation technology included larger cabin-class aircraft that allowed medical personnel to move around more and provide better care for patients. Pressurization made it possible to safely move more critically ill and injured patients than had been feasible before. One highly visible Mercy Flights initiative was the incorporation of neonatal transport systems—with the capability to provide heat, suction, oxygen, resuscitation, and vital monitoring for a newborn—into their services, saving the lives of many small and vulnerable infants born in the smaller hospitals throughout the region.

While it was not within its original mission, in 1992, Mercy Flights took on the responsibility for a countywide ground ambulance system when smaller commercial services cut back their service areas, refused services to patients with low resources, or were getting out of the business. (Ashland and Rogue River still maintain ambulances operated by their city governments.) Currently, Mercy Flights ground ambulances transport approximately 85 percent of patients in the valley.

As the region developed and FAA regulations changed, landing fixed-wing planes on highways and remote fields was prohibitive, so there arose a need for a helicopter operation. After initially leasing services from a local company for over 20 years, and with helicopter transports growing to over 200 per year, Mercy Flights bought its first helicopter in 2015. When they acquired the 2014 Bell 407GX, Mercy Flights also assumed complete responsibility for its maintenance and pilot training.

This book tells the story of how the region felt ownership for Mercy Flights, how the company later expanded to include a ground ambulance system and helicopters, and how it has continuously adapted to meet the ever-changing medical needs and health care access issues of the Southern Oregon/Northern California area.

As Michael E. Burrill Jr., current Mercy Flights board chairman, said, "Preparing our facilities and our organization for the ever-changing future of health care is our ongoing commitment. Mercy Flights will always be on the forefront of technology and patient care. Providing caring customer service along with premium medical treatment and transport at a reasonable cost will always be the number one mission for Mercy Flights."

One

MEETING A NEED

Located on the border of Southern Oregon and Northern California, the scenic Rogue Valley was the site of rapid population growth after World War II. Soldiers stationed in the region for training during World War II returned to the beautiful location to take advantage of the outdoor lifestyle, the moderate climate, and the welcoming environment they had experienced during their time in Medford and its surrounding small cities and towns.

These new residents brought with them a broad range of skills—many of them acquired during wartime—and were eager to participate in community solutions to emerging problems. No one could have predicted the sudden onset of the 1949 polio epidemic or the impact it would have on local populations residing far from complex medical treatment and rehabilitation facilities.

Rogue Valley residents—who generally valued their distance from "the big cities" of Portland, San Francisco, and even Eugene—were shocked to recognize the dangers of a six-hour emergency transport on a winding two-lane highway to the nearest iron lung in Eugene, which was over 100 miles away. Several well-known polio-stricken residents did not survive the trip or had their health permanently compromised because of this six-hour delay. Many were especially concerned about the young children who had contracted the disease. The community was upset. While they valued their two small hospitals and the trusted doctors in their medical community, there was widespread interest in a bigger solution.

Fortunately, George Milligan, a young FAA control tower operator—and pilot—had an idea. Allying with *Medford Mail Tribune* editor Eric Allen, Milligan proposed a volunteer air ambulance service with its first plane purchased through community donations. Highly skilled former military pilots would fly the planes, nurses and doctors would oversee the medical care, and an influential board of directors made up of community leaders would support the fledgling service. Mercy Flights was born.

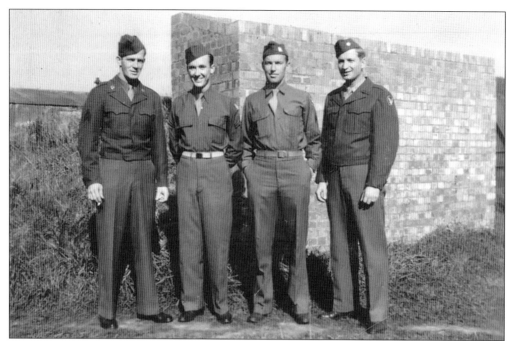

Trained as a civilian control tower operator in 1942, Mercy Flights founder George Milligan joined the US Army Air Corps in July 1944 as one of the first radar operators and technicians. He was assigned to England with a specialized group of radar experts with the long-term goal of supporting the Allies in their invasion of Europe on D-Day. After the invasion, they were reassigned to Paris to support the Army Air Corps and British pilots as the war wound down but the air fighting continued. Here, Milligan (third from left) is shown in front of barracks in Europe.

This CAA (Civilian Aeronautics Administration) paperwork details Milligan's assignments to the Medford Tower. As Mercy Flights grew and became increasingly visible both locally and nationally as America's first not-for-profit air ambulance service, there was increasing tension between Milligan's role in his federal job and his role as the leader of Mercy Flights. Several major attempts were made by the CAA and, later, the FAA to relocate Milligan to another community and a less visible role. However, interventions by community leaders and Oregon's Congressional delegation kept these transfers from occurring.

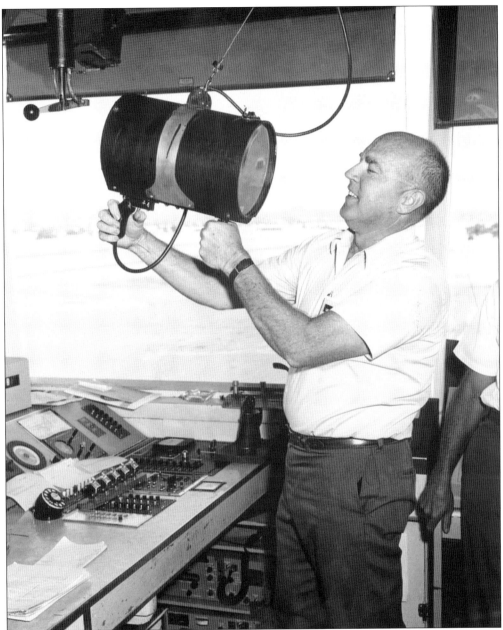

Born in Missouri and raised in Southern California, Mercy Flights founder George Milligan learned to fly at the Burbank, California, airport (now known as the Bob Hope Airport) at age 16. He was trained in Seattle as an air traffic controller by the Civil Aeronautics Administration (CAA) and was assigned to the Medford Tower prior to joining the Army Air Corps as a radarman in World War II. After returning from service in Britain and France, Milligan came back to Medford and the Medford Tower, where he is pictured in 1947. Milligan was an active and well-known pilot in the community when he founded Mercy Flights in 1949. (Photograph by Kenn Knackstedt.)

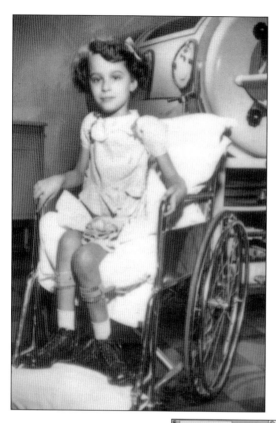

In the late 1940s and early 1950s, before the polio vaccine was available in 1955, polio was a major disease affecting children and adults. At the height of the polio epidemic in 1952, nearly 60,000 cases (with more than 3,000 deaths) were reported in the United States alone. Since polio was spread through water and food supplies, concern about the epidemic resulted in the closures of swimming pools and resort areas as well as the widespread use of public health isolation protocols discouraging public events. Rapid access to advanced medical care was crucial for survival in the most complex cases. Mercy Flights demonstrated the importance of this care.

Located on the Oregon-California border, Medford, Oregon, is a regional center for business, health care, and tourism. The nearest other urban centers and large hospitals are in Eugene (166 miles away), San Francisco (363 miles away), and Portland (274 miles away). The small communities of the Oregon coast, such as Gold Beach, are 150 miles away over a treacherous mountain range. Mercy Flights was created to minimize the time and trauma that sick and injured patients could incur on long and painful ground ambulance trips, which not uncommonly resulted in the death of the patient. (Courtesy of d-maps.com.)

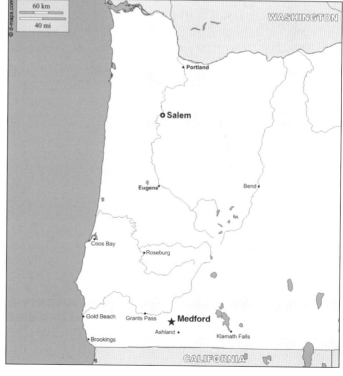

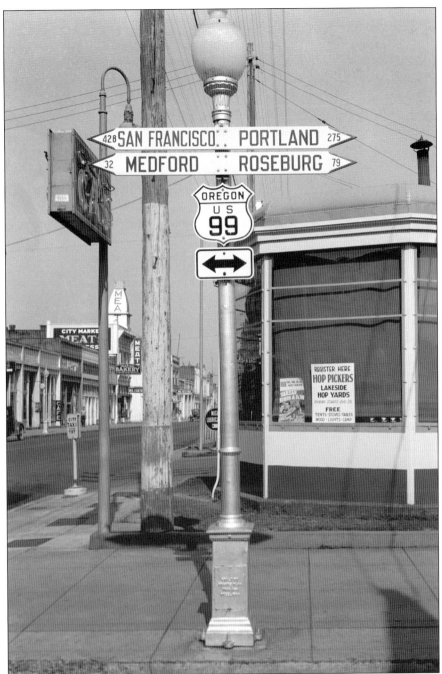

The construction of Interstate 5—the highway running the length of the West Coast through California, Oregon, and Washington—started in the mid-1950s and was not completed until 1966. Prior to that, car travel in and out of Southern Oregon primarily happened on US Route 99, later known as the Pacific Coast Highway. The two-lane highway wound through towns along the way, making for slow travel. This road sign in Grants Pass, Oregon, shows the distance to San Francisco (428 miles), Medford (32 miles), Portland (275 miles), and Roseburg (79 miles). (Photograph by Dorothea Lange; courtesy of Farm Security Administration.)

FORM ACA-500 (12-19-46) PART C	DEPARTMENT OF COMMERCE CIVIL AERONAUTICS ADMINISTRATION BILL OF SALE	FORM APPROVED BUDGET BUREAU NO. 41-R889

FOR AND IN CONSIDERATION OF $ 10.00 and other considerations / THE UNDERSIGNED OWNER OF THE FULL LEGAL AND BENEFICIAL TITLE OF THE AIRCRAFT DESCRIBED AS FOLLOWS:

AIRCRAFT MAKE	SERIAL NO.	CAA REGISTRATION NO.
Cessna UC 78 B	5556	NC 67185

DOES THIS **5th** DAY OF **October**, 19 **48** HEREBY SELL, GRANT, TRANSFER AND DELIVER ALL OF HIS RIGHT, TITLE AND INTEREST IN AND TO SUCH AIRCRAFT UNTO:

NAME OF PURCHASER
MERCY FLIGHTS, INC.

ADDRESS OF PURCHASER (*Street and number, city, zone and state*)
BROPHY BLDG., MEDFORD, OREGON

AND TO **its** EXECUTORS, ADMINISTRATORS AND ASSIGNS, TO HAVE AND TO HOLD SINGULARLY, THE SAID AIRCRAFT FOREVER, AND CERTIFIES THAT SAME IS NOT SUBJECT TO ANY MORTGAGE OR OTHER ENCUMBRANCE EXCEPT:

TYPE OF ENCUMBRANCE	AMOUNT	DATE
None	None	

IN FAVOR OF
No one

IN TESTIMONY WHEREOF **I** HAVE SET **My** HAND AND SEAL THIS **5th** DAY OF **October**, 19**48**

SIGNATURE OF SELLER
[signature]

TITLE OF SELLER
President – Coast Air Ambulance

FOR (*Name of corporation, partnership*)
Coast Air Ambulance

ACKNOWLEDGMENT

STATE OF **California**

COUNTY OF **Alameda**

ON THIS **5th** DAY OF **October**, 19 **48** BEFORE ME PERSONALLY APPEARED THE ABOVE-NAMED SELLER, TO ME KNOWN TO BE THE PERSON DESCRIBED IN AND WHO EXECUTED THE FOREGOING BILL OF SALE, AND ACKNOWLEDGED THAT HE EXECUTED THE SAME AS HIS FREE ACT AND DEED. GIVEN UNDER MY HAND AND OFFICIAL SEAL THE DAY AND YEAR ABOVE WRITTEN.

NOTARY PUBLIC — MY COMMISSION EXPIRES
[signature] Dec. 17, 1950
Seal

READ INSTRUCTIONS ON REVERSE SIDE CAREFULLY

A-3319-0(2)+

RETAINED BY PURCHASER – USE TYPEWRITER

As documented in this bill of sale, Mercy Flights was able to purchase a used Twin Cessna to serve as its first plane prior to the formal incorporation of the service. Community fundraisers by schoolchildren, service clubs, and churches raised money to upgrade the plane and outfit it for air ambulance use.

Mercy Flights' first plane is shown below as it looked when it was purchased (prior to its refurbishing and modification for use as an air ambulance). The Twin Cessna became the backdrop for the first photographs of Mercy Flights "in action," including pictures of the inauguration of the service with a dedication of the plane and multiple photographs of patients with ambulance crews, pilots, nurses, and family members.

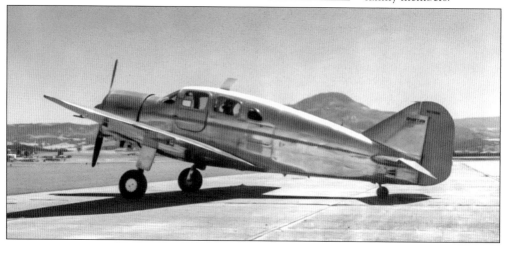

Jeanette Thatcher Marshall, the first female attorney in Medford, Oregon, served as secretary for Mercy Flights from its 1949 beginning through the 1980s. She provided valuable advice, careful documentation, and important connections to other members of the Southern Oregon legal community when their expertise was needed. (Courtesy of Marie Garsjo.)

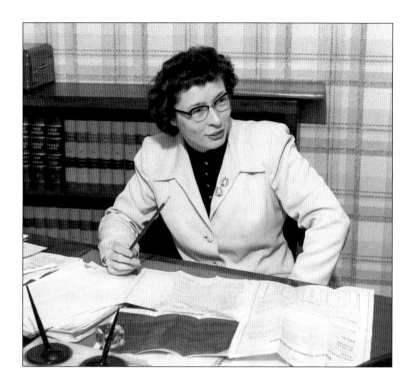

Articles of Incorporation

OF

MERCY FLIGHTS, INCORPORATED

We, George E. Milligan, C. I. Drummond and Jeannette E. Thatcher

whose names are hereunto subscribed, desiring to form a corporation under and by virtue of Chapter 462, Oregon Laws, 1941, providing for the creation of nonprofit corporations, do hereby associate ourselves together and make and execute in triplicate the following articles of incorporation, to wit:

ARTICLE I

The name assumed by this corporation and by which it shall be known is

MERCY FLIGHTS, INC.

and its duration shall be perpetual.

On August 24, 1949, Jeanette Marshall drafted and then submitted Mercy Flights' Articles of Incorporation to the State of Oregon.

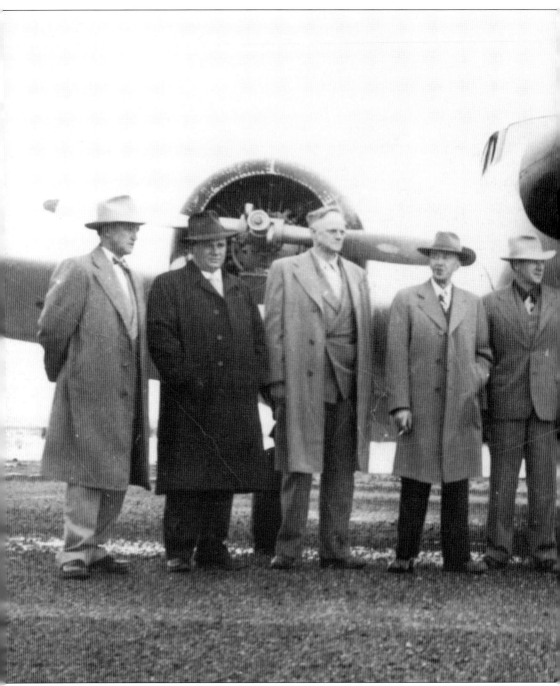

Mercy Flights' first board of directors is pictured in January 1950 on a rainy day at the Medford Airport with the first Mercy Flights plane. This carefully chosen, community-focused group volunteered to provide guidance and leadership to the fledgling organization. Pictured from left to right are board members Dr. L. Paul Walker (dentist), Frank Perl (mortician), R.A. Skinner (owner of a local car dealership), Harold Frye (a small-business owner), Vern Smith (local president

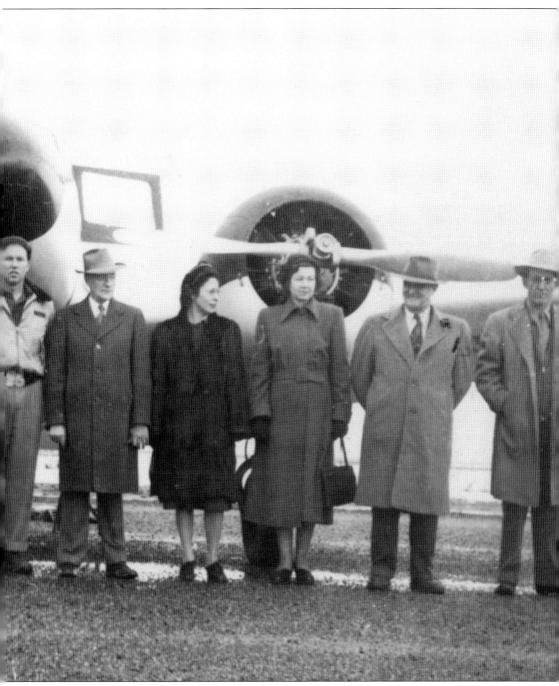

of the National Foundation for Infantile Paralysis), George Milligan (chairman and founder of Mercy Flights), Rev. Harry Hansen, Jeanette Thatcher (lawyer), Mrs. Stephen G. Nye (representing orchardists), Mayor Diamond Flynn, and Sheriff Howard Gault. The board members not pictured are Eric Allen, editor of the Medford Mail Tribune; Seth Bullis, a businessman; and Dr. C.I. Drummond, a local physician. (Courtesy of Mercy Flights and the Southern Oregon Historical Society.)

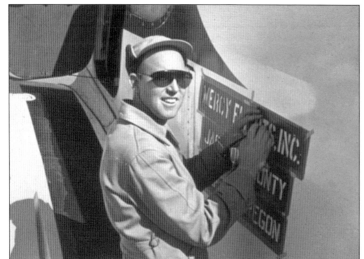

George Milligan welcomed each of the new planes as they came on board. He was also proud to stencil "Mercy Flights, Inc." on each plane.

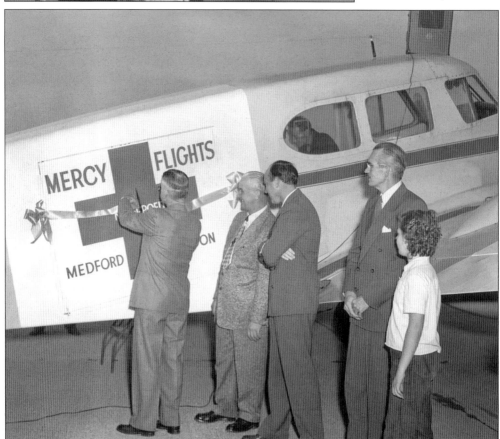

Southern Oregon residents successfully raised the $3,000 necessary to refurbish and upgrade Mercy Flights' first plane, a Twin Cessna Bobcat. The community celebration included a ribbon-cutting ceremony for the new door of the plane. From left to right in this photograph are Gov. Douglas McKay (cutting the ribbon), Medford mayor Diamond Flynn, George Milligan, and two unidentified people. (Photograph by Kenn Knackstedt.)

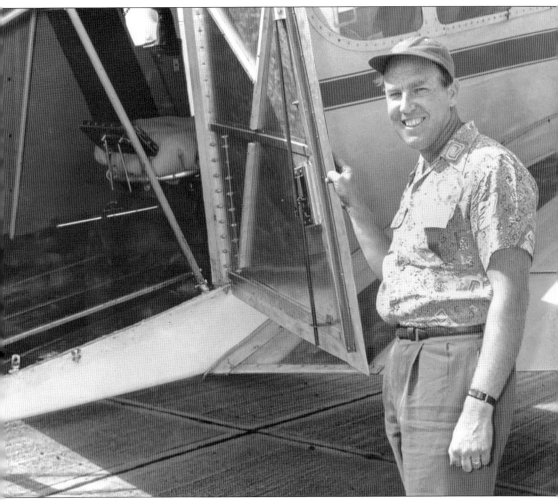

Before the new Mercy Flights planes could be fully utilized, each one required individualized door modifications and expansions necessary for the loading and unloading of the patient and the stretcher. The final step in this process was FAA approval. In addition to serving as the leader of Mercy Flights, George Milligan also designed and engineered each of these modifications and is shown here with the expanded door on Mercy Flights' first plane. (Photograph by Kenn Knackstedt.)

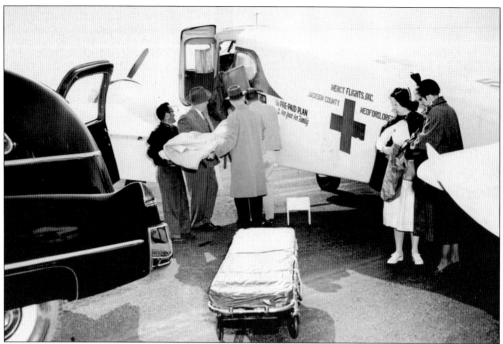

In this photograph taken at the Roseburg Airport on March 26, 1952, a patient is being loaded—with difficulty—into the a Mercy Flights plane prior to the addition of a larger door. The patient's sister-in-law and a Mercy Flights nurse are at right. (Courtesy of Mercy Flights and the Southern Oregon Historical Society.)

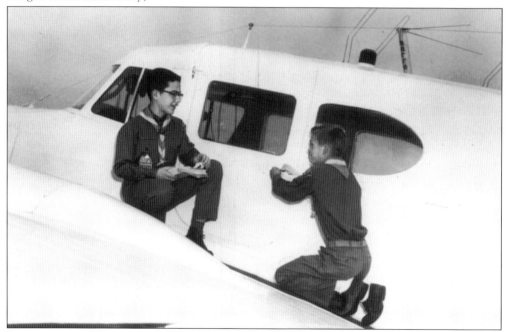

In recognition of the many community contributions that raised funds to purchase the first Mercy Flights Twin Cessna, these two scouts were allowed to paint logos and apply stencils on the historic plane. (Courtesy of Mercy Flights and the Southern Oregon Historical Society.)

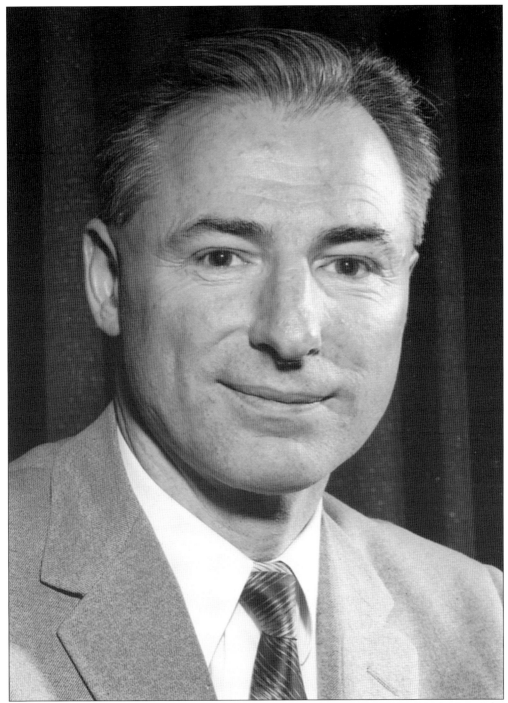

George Flanagan, along with Jeanette Marshall and Eric Allen, served as the foundation of the Mercy Flights board of directors for many years. A local lumberman, Flanagan was the president of Elk Lumber Company and was extensively involved in the community at all levels, gave outstanding financial advice, and brought other leaders of the area's lumber industry on board. (Courtesy of the *Medford Mail Tribune*.)

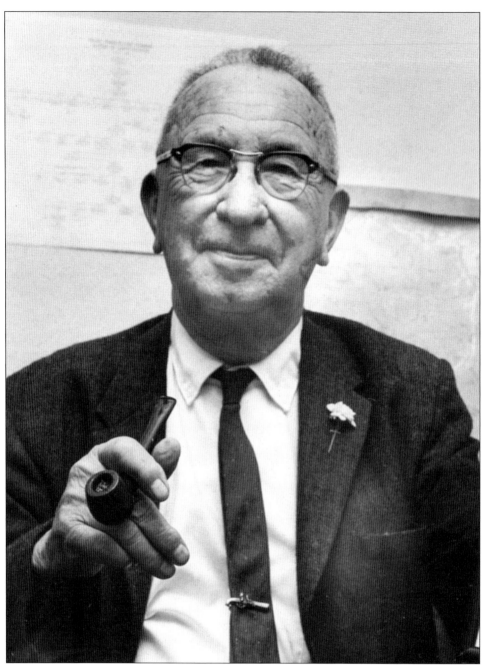

Seth Bullis, one of Mercy Flights' original board members, was an example of a great choice to guide a developing community organization. A well-known businessman who was heavily involved in the community, Bullis was a member of the Masons, the Elks Club, and the Presbyterian church. His businesses included his ownership of the Sterling Mine, the oldest placer mine in Southern Oregon. Later, he served as an organizer and treasurer for the Southern Oregon Lumber company and established the Rogue River Valley Canning Company, where he served as president. Known for recognizing needs and opportunities, Bullis consistently provided Mercy Flights with valuable business advice. (Courtesy of the *Medford Mail Tribune*.)

Complex care of patients with respiratory complications stemming from polio required iron lungs—sometimes for the patient's entire life—and 24-hour nursing care. The public was fascinated with these complex machines, which provided a quick visual image of the devastating disease and motivated people to adopt and comply with public health and safety measures. (Courtesy of OHSU Historical Collections & Archives.)

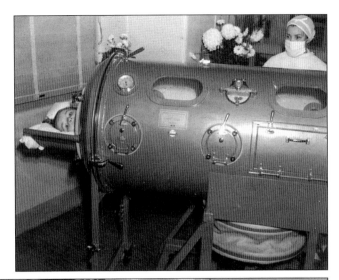

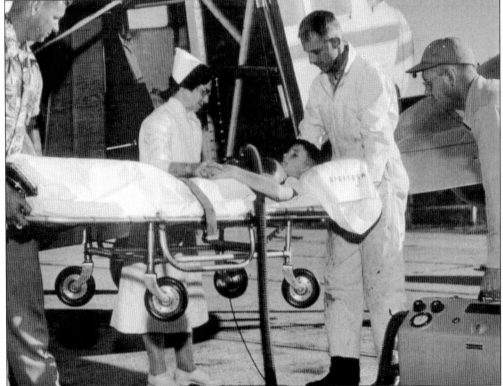

This early-1950s photograph shows a young polio patient with a portable respirator, which replaced the bulky and confining iron lungs used during the early days of the polio epidemic. The actual respirator is visible in the lower right corner of this image. While polio treatments improved, many patients were hospitalized for years as they regained their strength, went through rehabilitation, and were trained in the use of crutches and other mobility devices. An interesting feature of this photograph is the "SPEBSQSA" (Society for the Preservation and Encouragement of Barber Shop Quartet Singing in America) label on the pillowcase; the SPEBSQSA conducted regular fundraisers to benefit Mercy Flights and made donations of linens and other medical equipment.

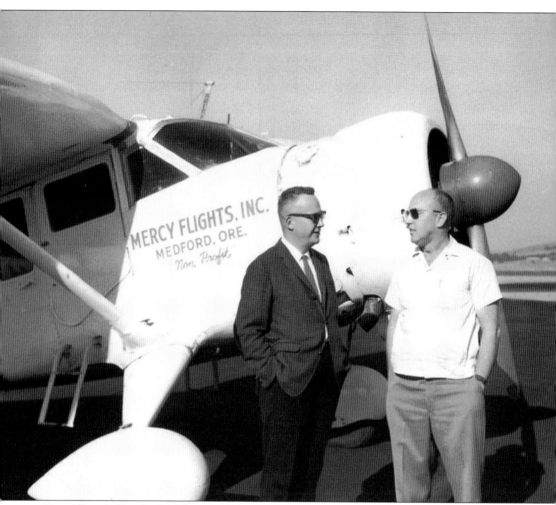

Eric Allen (left), editor of the *Medford Mail Tribune,* is pictured with George Milligan next to a Mercy Flights Stinson Reliant, which was useful for landing on small and remote airstrips. Allen's involvement in the creation and sustainability of Mercy Flights was a key factor in the success of the service. Allen—who provided important stories about the need for Mercy Flights, strategized about next steps for the organization, created linkages with community leaders, and served as Mercy Flights' treasurer until 1985—was a confidant of Milligan in both good and difficult times.

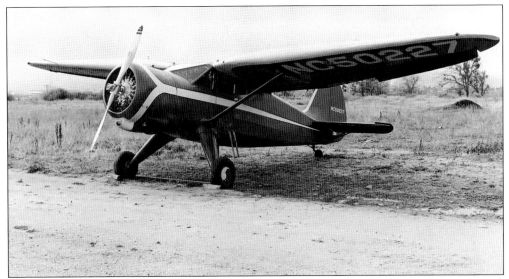

A single-engine workhorse with the flexibility to utilize small landing strips, this Mercy Flights Stinson was affectionately named "Rudolph… The Red Nosed Stinson." The plane is shown here at a small rural airstrip. (Courtesy of Mercy Flights and the Southern Oregon Historical Society.)

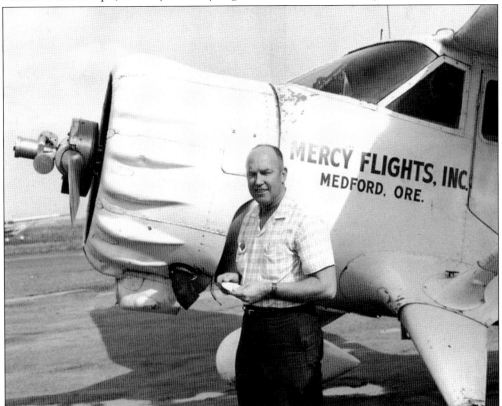

George Milligan was especially proud of Mercy Flights' Stinson Reliant because of its ability to land in remote areas. Mercy Flights' volunteer pilots valued time spent in the resilient plane, which was reportedly fun to fly.

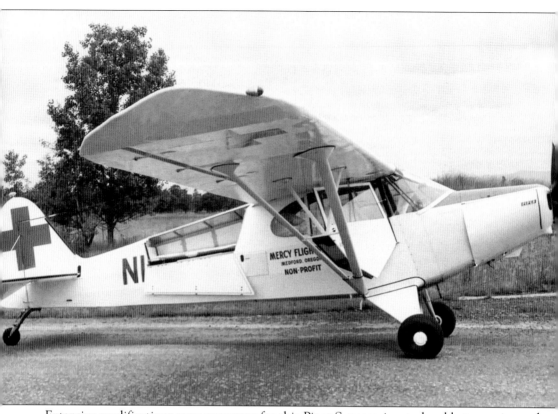

Extensive modifications were necessary for this Piper Supercruiser to be able to receive and transport a patient and his/her stretcher. This photograph clearly shows the door that was cut into the side of the aircraft.

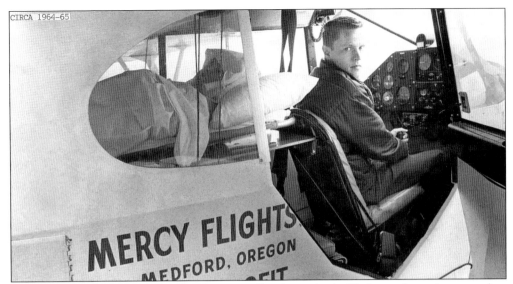

All of the original Mercy Flights planes were small and completely filled once the patient, stretcher, and nurse were on board. This side view of the Mercy Flights Piper Supercruiser, nicknamed "Band-Aid," shows how tight it could be.

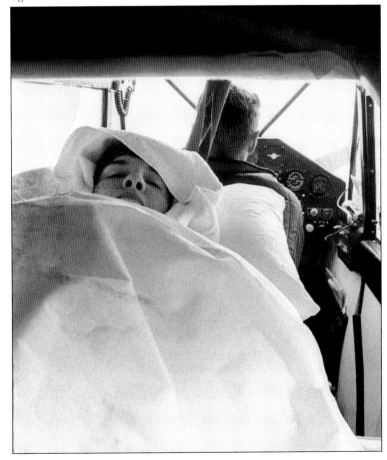

Early Mercy Flights planes were small and cramped. This picture of a patient and a copilot in the Mercy Flights Supercruiser shows the intimacy of the experience. If needed, a nurse could be tightly packed into the small space behind the pilot after everyone else was on board.

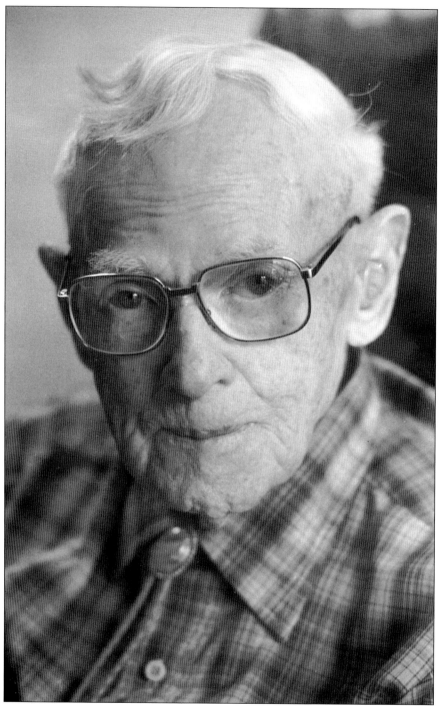

Original Mercy Flights board of directors member R.A. Skinner owned the local Buick dealership and encouraged his fellow businessmen to support Mercy Flights. Skinner's son Lon served with George Milligan in the Army Air Corps in England in World War II and was a major influence on Milligan's decision to return to Medford to work for the CAA after the war. (Courtesy of the *Medford Mail Tribune*.)

Two

COMMUNITY ACTION AND LEADERSHIP

Community leaders mobilized to promote Mercy Flights through fundraising, devising communications strategies, streamlining a subscription/membership process, and offering legal and technical advice.

The Mercy Flights board represented a cross section of the power structure in the Rogue Valley. In addition to their direct involvement on what was initially a time-consuming board, each member also brought with them their access to a wide range of colleagues and friends. Their influence reached deeply into the community, and they all knew they were expected to capitalize on this reach.

Medford mayor Diamond Flynn brought on board his peers in Ashland, Grants Pass, Central Point, Jacksonville, Phoenix, and Talent. Harry Hanson, minister at the First Presbyterian Church in Medford, reached out to his religious counterparts. George Flanagan, president of Elk Lumber Company, worked with logging and lumber company leaders for financial support and eventually coordinated lumber donations for the construction of Mercy Flights' first hangar. Lawyer Jeanette Marshall kept her legal colleagues updated on Mercy Flights' issues and subsequently enlisted them in helping to resolve complex legal issues with governmental agencies like the Federal Aviation Administration (FAA). *Medford Mail Tribune* editor Eric Allen provided strategic advice to founder George Milligan and arranged media coverage not just in newspapers but also on both radio and newly developing television stations.

The sustainability of Mercy Flights required a stable financial structure. As the board grappled with this issue, Milligan proposed a subscription plan that would provide medical transportation when needed to families covered by an annual subscription. The board enthusiastically supported this strategy and created community subscription drives, making subscriptions readily available in local offices and businesses and encouraging employers to provide subscriptions as a benefit of employment.

Another way the board worked to balance the Mercy Flights budget was by obtaining surplus military aircraft. Twin-engine Beechcraft were identified as being appropriate planes for air ambulance use. While the members of the organization were aware that acquiring these aircraft would be a complex process, no one knew that it would literally take an act of Congress to transfer these planes to Mercy Flights through a partnership with Rogue Valley Memorial Hospital. The Oregon Congressional Delegation sprang into action, and based on their success, Mercy Flights received two planes from US Air Force surplus on July 30, 1959.

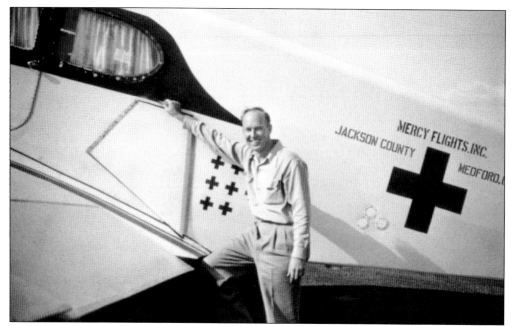

Founder George Milligan is smiling proudly next to the first Mercy Flights' plane. In keeping with the military experience of most of the volunteer pilots at Mercy Flights, the original plan was to paint a small red cross on each plane to signify each successful mission. This soon became unrealistic as the number of flights increased; however, the idea was a good one in terms of visually depicting the service's growth.

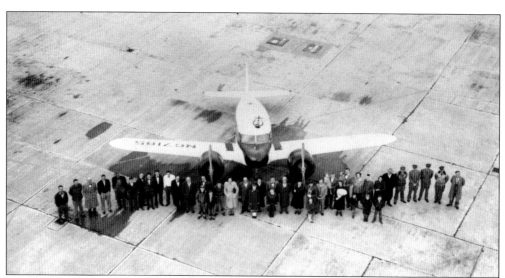

In February 1951, a group of 45 people—including leaders, pilots, nurses, airport personnel, and members of the SPEBSQSA (Society for the Preservation and Encouragement of Barber Shop Quartet Singing in America)—lined up to celebrate the 45th patient carried by Mercy Flights. (Courtesy of Mercy Flights and the Southern Oregon Historical Society.)

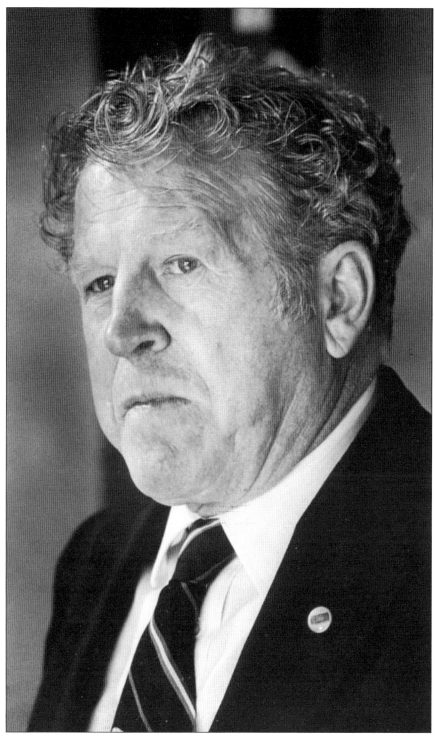

Early Mercy Flights board member Eugene F. Burrill owned a lumber company in White City, situated on the outskirts of Medford. Burrill was also a pilot and flew missions and rescue flights for Mercy Flights into small and remote communities. (Courtesy of the *Medford Mail Tribune*.)

YOU

ARE

MERCY FLIGHTS

No Other public service organization is so completely owned by those it serves. $5.00 a year per family entitles you to the best air ambulance service in the world, FREE within a 400 mile radius of Medford, for medical emergences.

Over 150 patients a year benefit from this life-saving service. If YOU never need it, your subscription has helped those less fortunate. New subscriptions and donations received at this time will go toward purchasing the government planes that have been loaned to Mercy Flights for the past several years. A more efficient and faster service to YOU will result.

Like the Oregon state motto, "She flies with her own wings," Mercy Flights depends for support on the people she serves — the residents of southern Oregon and northern California.

PROTECT YOURSELF AND YOUR NEIGHBOR FOR ONLY—

$5

A YEAR PER FAMILY

•

Join Today!

Get Application Blanks at:
- COOS-CURRY ELECTRIC (Gold Beach and Port Orford)
- BILL & LENA'S MARKET
- BUFFINGTON MOTORS
- BROOKINGS SUPPLY
- CURRY COUNTY REPORTER

MERCY FLIGHTS, INC.

P. O. Box 522   Medford, Oregon

If in doubt, ask one of the 1400 patients whose lives have been saved.

GOLD BEACH FLYING CLUB

Mercy Flights implemented subscription fees in May 1951. These were initially priced at $2 per family per year, then increased to $4 ($2 for an individual) in March 1955 and raised to $5 per year ($3 for an individual) in 1959. The subscriptions were sold at community businesses at a time when most people still paid their bills in person. In addition, subscriptions were available at local events including county fairs, parades, picnics, and school sports events. Employers such as lumber companies bought subscriptions for their workers as an employee benefit. In addition, locally sponsored air shows were presented at the region's small airports to promote and support Mercy Flights.

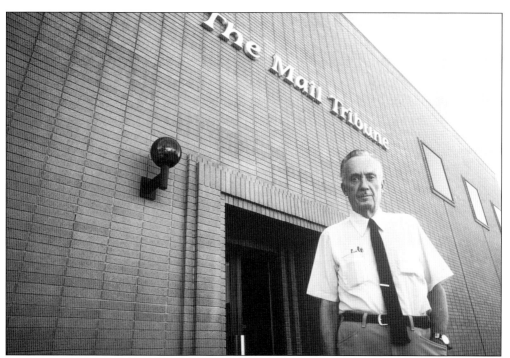

Editor Eric Allen is pictured outside the headquarters of the *Medford Mail Tribune*. Allen and George Milligan were friends and colleagues and worked together to create consistent strategic plans and messages about Mercy Flights. They met frequently at Allen's office in downtown Medford.

Mercy Flights was funded entirely by community contributions. A donation program in which schoolchildren collected coins in empty milk cartons contributed to the purchase of the first plane. Mercy Flights later transitioned to a subscription-funded service in which a person could pay a small subscription each year in exchange for emergency medical transportation to higher levels of care if needed. This contributed advertisement in the *Ashland Daily Tidings* promotes Mercy Flights subscriptions and also shows off the newly arrived and refurbished Twin Beechcrafts obtained by Mercy Flights and Rogue Valley Memorial Hospital from World War II Air Force surplus. (Courtesy of the *Ashland Daily Tidings*.)

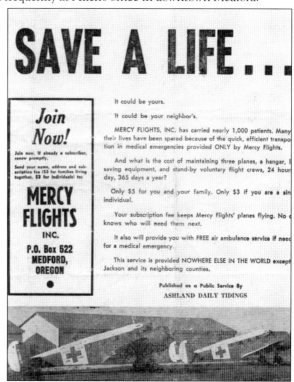

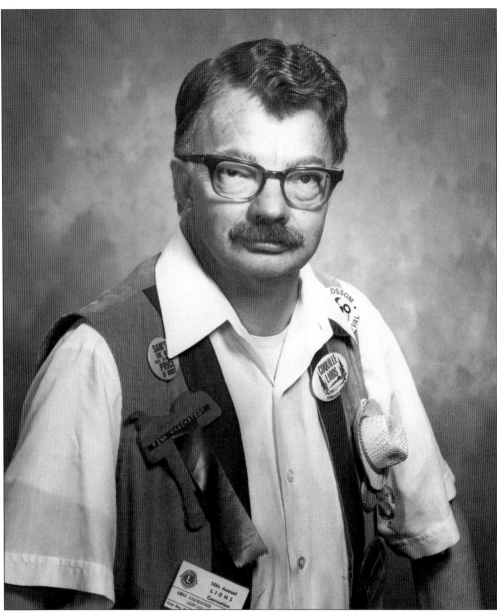

At a time when local commercial photographers needed a special focus to survive, Medford photographer Kenn Knackstedt was attracted to the aviation culture of the Medford Airport and hung out at Mercy Flights to document the challenges facing a nonprofit air ambulance service. Collected in his "Sky Billy Series," Knackstedt's subjects include pilots, patients, and planes. Knackstedt's photographs are interspersed throughout this publication. (Courtesy of the *Medford Mail Tribune*.)

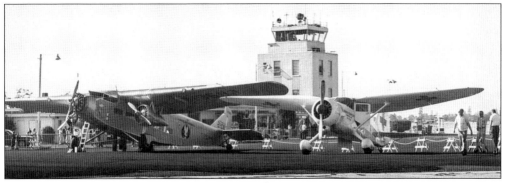

Air shows were major community activities in the 1950s, serving to promote aviation, raise funds, and get schoolchildren interested in the future. Mercy Flights' first single-engine plane, the Stinson Reliant (at right), is pictured at a Medford airshow next to a visiting Ford Tri-motor with the newly constructed Medford Tower in the background.

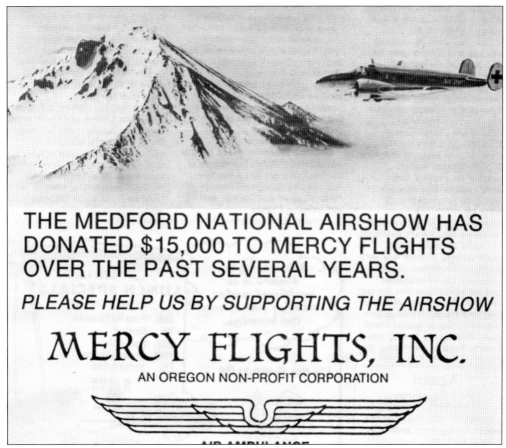

The *Medford Mail Tribune* regularly contributed space to promote Mercy Flights and its fundraising/subscription initiatives. This advertisement thanks the Medford National Airshow organizers for their donations in support of Mercy Flights.

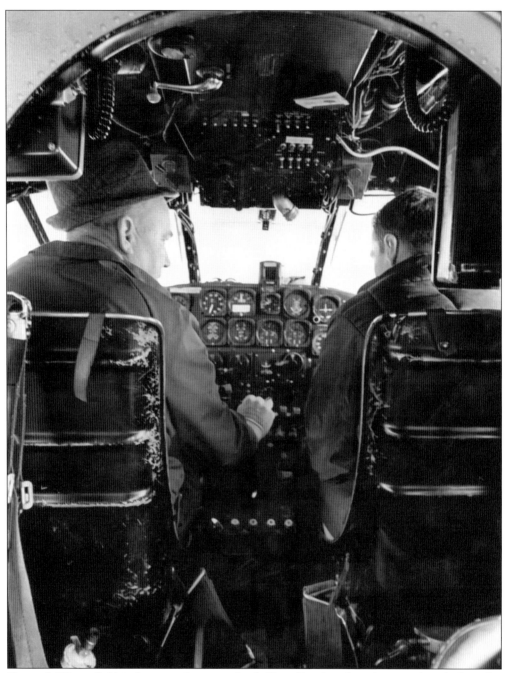

George Milligan (left) is shown at the controls of a Twin Beechcraft with an unidentified copilot in the early stages of the plane's remake into a civilian air ambulance. Throughout his career, Milligan was an instructor and role model for many younger pilots, many of whom eventually flew for Mercy Flights.

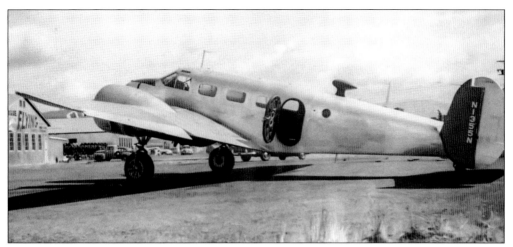

Two Twin Beechcrafts obtained from the US Air Force in 1951 were picked up by Mercy Flights pilots at a storage depot in Arizona. Acquisition of these planes—for $1.50 per plane—required the joint sponsorship of Rogue Valley Memorial Hospital and an act of Congress. The first plane is shown upon its arrival in Medford.

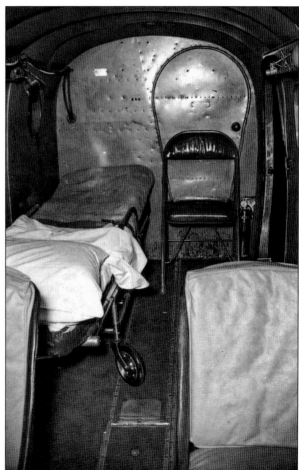

The two surplus Air Force Twin Beechcraft had been used to transport supplies and were pretty basic inside. This is early interior photograph of one of the first Beechcraft shows the stretcher and a "moveable" seat for the nurse. Another seat closer to the pilots and facing backward toward the patient and the nurse could be used by the patient's spouse or friend.

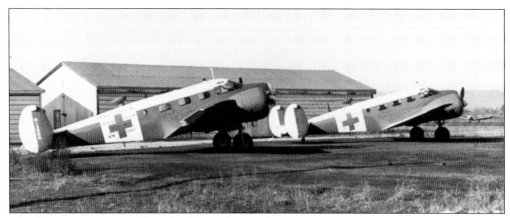

The first two Twin Beechcraft planes obtained from Air Force surplus are pictured newly painted, modified, and reconfigured for Mercy Flights service. (Courtesy of the Southern Oregon Historical Society.)

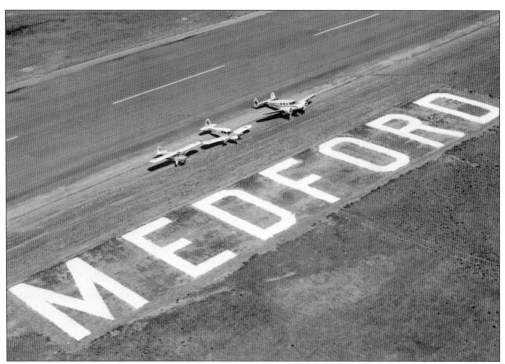

Three of the first Mercy Flights planes are shown lined up on the ramp at the Medford Airport for a photo opportunity for Kenn Knackstedt. (Courtesy of the Southern Oregon Historical Society.)

A major sustainability issue for Mercy Flights was keeping its planes protected. The first planes could be kept in borrowed hangar space, but larger planes and their equipment needed larger buildings. In keeping with their tradition of recruiting community volunteers, Mercy Flights ran this advertisement in collaboration with the *Medford Mail Tribune* on May 6, 1959, in search of carpenters to build a new hangar with donated lumber and supplies.

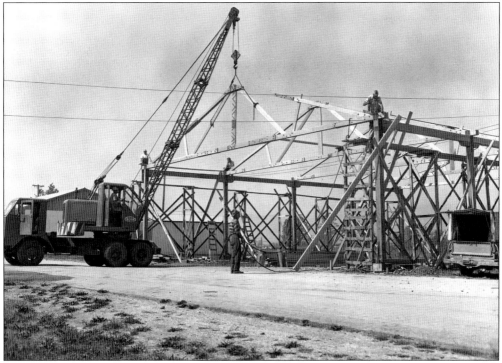

After the organization acquired the first two Mercy Flights planes, the next step was to build a hangar to protect them. Community fundraisers, donations from lumber companies, volunteer labor from loggers and construction workers, and food (provided by women's clubs) for volunteers made it happen. (Photograph by Kenn Knackstedt.)

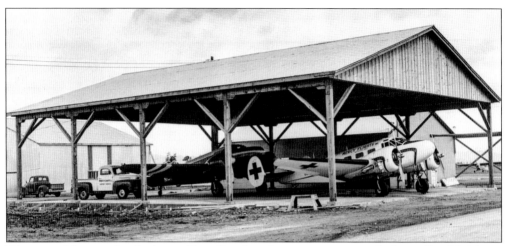

The second hangar for the larger Twin Beechcrafts was open air, with the walls added later. Two of the early Mercy Flights planes are shown safe and dry in their new home. (Photograph by Kenn Knackstedt.)

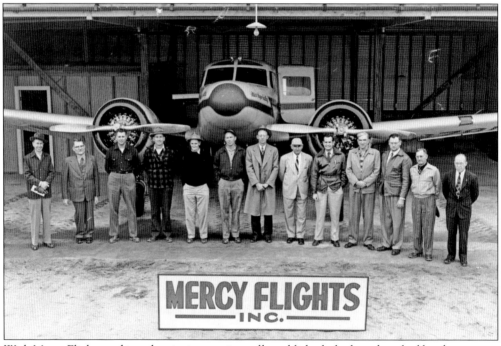

With Mercy Flights and its subscription service well established, the board worked hard to protect the planes with the first Mercy Flights hangar at the Medford Airport. Community members who donated time and materials are pictured here. From left to right are W.E. Brooks, Homer Bell, Lee Flink, Elmo Viar, Bart Shepherd, George Milligan, Al Nielson, Roy Ganfield, Jack Edmonds, L.V. Ward, Joel Elkins, Clyde Richmond, and Al Miller. (Courtesy of the Southern Oregon Historical Society.)

The transfer of Air Force surplus Twin Beechcraft planes to Mercy Flights required upgrading, repainting, and significant mechanical support. Here, two mechanics for Mercy Flights are working on one of the new planes shortly after it was repainted. (Courtesy of the Southern Oregon Historical Society.)

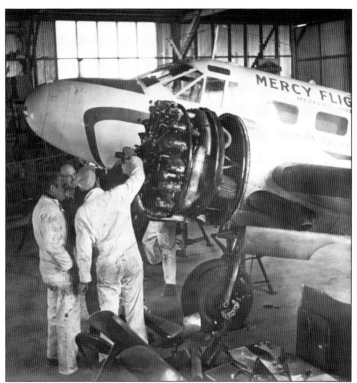

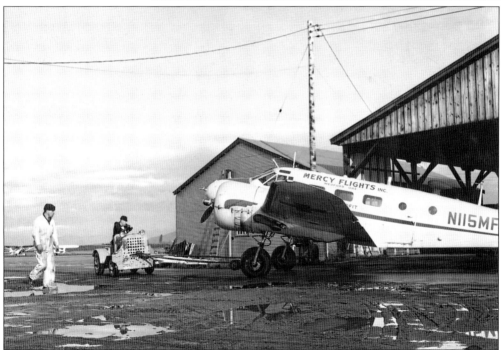

Moving the large planes in and out of the hangar was not easy. Fortunately, as a nonprofit organization, Mercy Flights was able to acquire other federal surplus equipment such as a special small tractor used to move their larger planes. (Photograph by Kenn Knackstedt.)

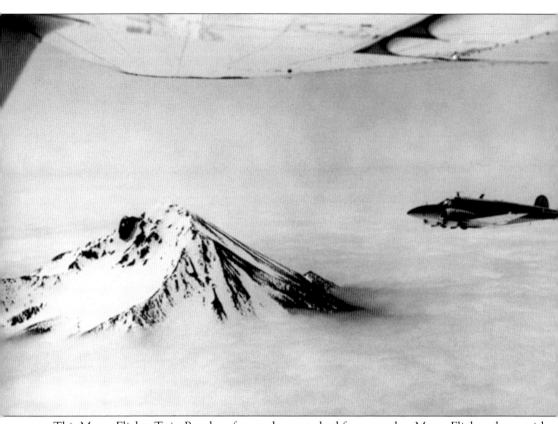

This Mercy Flights Twin Beechcraft was photographed from another Mercy Flights plane, with Southern Oregon's Mt. McLaughlin in the background.

Three

SETTLING IN

As Mercy Flights was building a diverse fleet and participating in a wide range of fundraising events, issues of federal governmental regulation were taking up more and more of the organization's time. At the simplest level, governmental review and approval were required for the structural modifications that had to be made to each newly acquired aircraft in order to allow stretchers and patients to be loaded into very small planes through unique new doors.

Prior to the creation of Mercy Flights, the only federal regulations even partially applicable to air ambulances governed air taxis. The specificity of these regulations was a major barrier to the creation of medical air transport services. In 1971, the FAA communicated to the Mercy Flights board their intention to apply air taxi rules to Mercy Flights. This ruling would potentially put Mercy Flights out of business by eliminating their nonprofit status and putting limits on their ability to fly in certain weather conditions and rescue situations. Mercy Flights immediately launched a strong opposition effort involving the community, the media, local mayors, and Oregon's congressional delegation.

Prestigious Medford attorney Otto Frohnmayer was enlisted to work with Mercy Flights lawyer and board member Jeanette Marshall on the case. In 1971, the FAA scheduled a hearing at the federal courthouse in Medford for Wednesday, October 20. It was a painful experience for everyone. The FAA quickly issued a ruling that the air taxi rules would be applied to Mercy Flights. Led by Sen. Mark Hatfield, the Oregon congressional delegation jumped into action, demanding a more thorough review of Mercy Flights. An FAA medical director was assigned to spend time in Medford and personally observe operations, flights, and patient transfers. He issued a positive report, including the recommendation that Mercy Flights serve as the model for other developing air ambulances. The FAA reversed their earlier ruling, and Mercy Flights continued operating.

In 1978, the FAA attempted to implement standards related to air ambulances that would have put Mercy Flights out of business. This time, Oregon senator Bob Packwood successfully led congressional opposition to support the development of a broader and less-specific regulatory environment to flexibly allow the air ambulance movement to develop and thrive. These federal interactions would continue throughout the history of Mercy Flights.

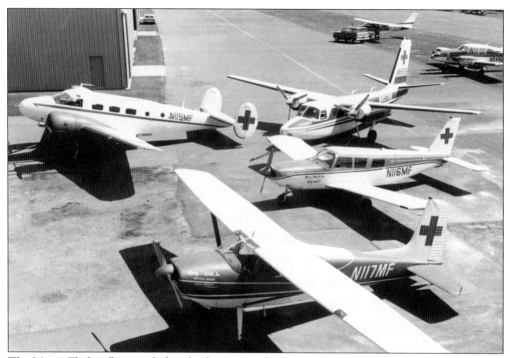

The Mercy Flights fleet, including both twin- and single-engine aircraft, is shown at the Mercy Flights hangar at the Medford Airport. This variety of airplanes allowed Mercy Flights to offer optimum service to a wide range of airports and airstrips in the region.

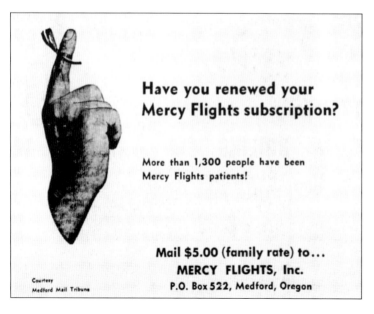

Have you renewed your Mercy Flights subscription?

More than 1,300 people have been Mercy Flights patients!

Mail $5.00 (family rate) to...
MERCY FLIGHTS, Inc.
P.O. Box 522, Medford, Oregon

The *Medford Mail Tribune* supported Mercy Flights through regular advertisements for the company's subscription campaigns.

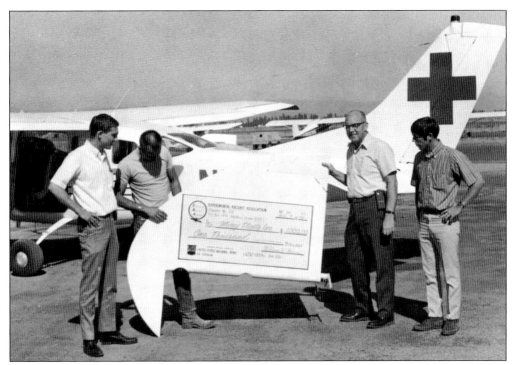

Local air shows were consistent fundraisers for Mercy Flights over the years. In 1970, the Experimental Aircraft Association (EAA) sponsored a show in recognition of Mercy Flights' 21 years of service. Shown presenting the donation check—which is enlarged and attached to the rudder of Mercy Flights' first plane—are, from left to right, Mercy Flights pilots and EAA officers Bill Warren and Gar Laviea, Mercy Flights founder George Milligan, and EAA officer Fred Quazzo.

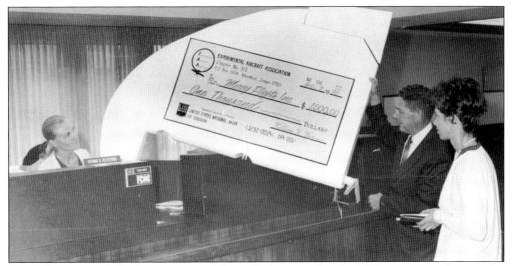

After the oversized check was given to Mercy Flights, people asked, "But can you take it to the bank?" Mercy Flights manager Diane Coash (far right) enjoyed the challenge of presenting the EAA donation for deposit to the Mercy Flights bank account.

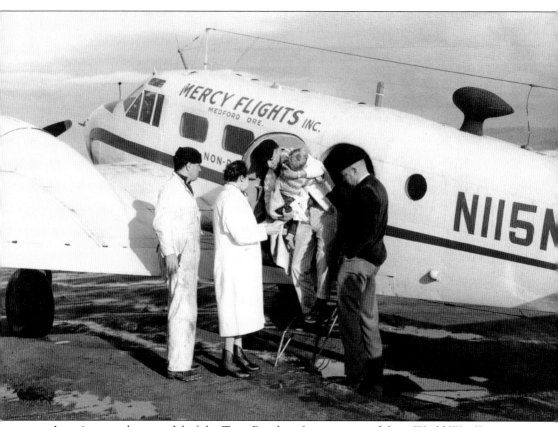

Iron Annie, a later model of the Twin Beechcraft, was acquired from World War II government surplus. She is shown here soon after she was moved to Medford.

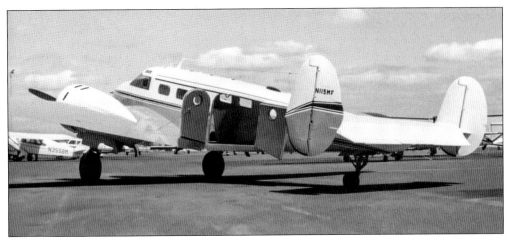

Relatively larger planes like Iron Annie, shown later in her career, also required door modifications so that patients could be quickly moved into and out of the air ambulance. Here, Iron Annie is shown with her modified doors opened.

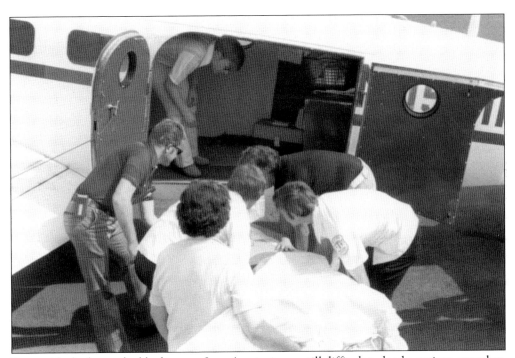

Even with the larger double doors on Iron Annie, it was still difficult to load a patient, stretcher, and supporting medical technology into an air ambulance.

DEPARTMENT OF TRANSPORTATION
FEDERAL AVIATION ADMINISTRATION

CERTIFIED MAIL - RETURN RECEIPT REQUESTED

NOTICE OF HEARING

SERVICE:

MERCY FLIGHTS, INC.
Box 522
Medford, Oregon 97501

GEORGE E. MILLIGAN
Chairman, Mercy Flights, Inc.
Box 522   and   1812 Archer Drive
Medford, Oregon 97501   Medford, Oregon 97501

GEORGE C. FLANAGAN
Vice Chairman
Mercy Flights, Inc.
Box 522   and   Ehrman Way
Medford, Oregon 97501   Medford, Oregon 97501

ERIC ALLEN, JR.
Treasurer, Mercy Flights, Inc. and   Medford Tribune
Box 522   P. O. Box 1108
Medford, Oregon 97501   Medford, Oregon 97501

JEANNETTE T. MARSHALL
Secretary, Mercy Flights, Inc. and   Brophy Building
Box 522   246 East 10th Street
Medford, Oregon 97501   Medford, Oregon 97501

In the Matter of the Federal Aviation Administration)
Investigation of Operations Conducted by Mercy Flights,)
Inc. without holding an Air Taxi Operator/Commercial)
Operator Certificate.)

Notice is hereby given, pursuant to Sections 313(c), 1002(b), and
1004 of the Federal Aviation Act of 1958, as amended, (49 U.S.C. 1354,
1482, and 1484), that the above entitled proceeding will be heard before
the undersigned and such members of the hearing panel as he may designate
on Wednesday, the 20th day of October 1971, beginning at 9:30 a.m. in the
Courtroom, Federal Building Courthouse, 6th and Holly, Medford, Oregon.

Dated this 20th day of September 1971.

JONATHAN HOWE
Regional Counsel

The Federal Aviation Administration (FAA) was always tracking Mercy Flights closely, because it was American's first not-for-profit community based air ambulance, and on September 20, 1971, they issued a notice of hearing to the officers of Mercy Flights. Their intent was to apply commercial air taxi rules to Mercy Flights and other similar air ambulance services, which would result in the removal of their not-for profit status, threatening their future.

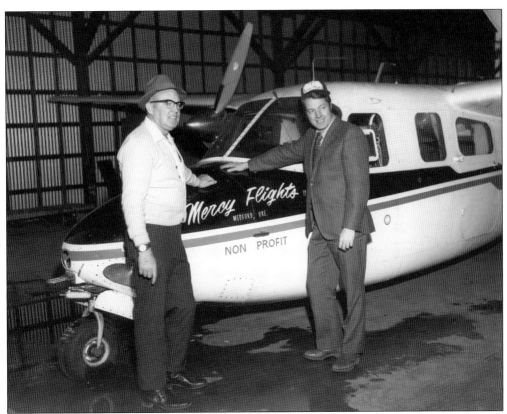

Local politicians from small cities and towns throughout Southern Oregon and Northern California were strong Mercy Flights supporters. Medford mayor William Singler (right), pictured here with George Milligan, was quick to respond to the notice from the FAA. (Courtesy of the Southern Oregon Historical Society.)

Medford mayor William Singler's letter to the FAA discussed the valuable contribution that Mercy Flights made to Medford and the surrounding region. He also announced a resolution in support of Mercy Flights that was quickly passed by the Medford City Council.

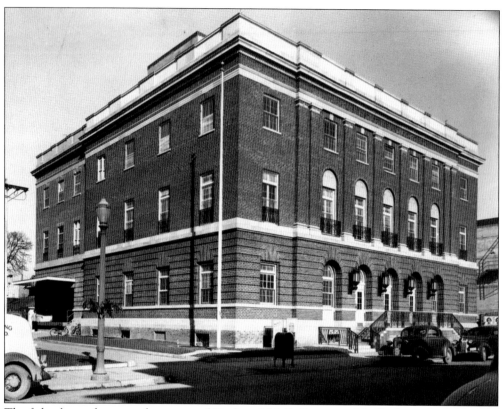

The federal courthouse at the corner of Sixth and Holly Streets in Medford was the setting for the FAA hearings regarding Mercy Flights. (Courtesy of the National Archives.)

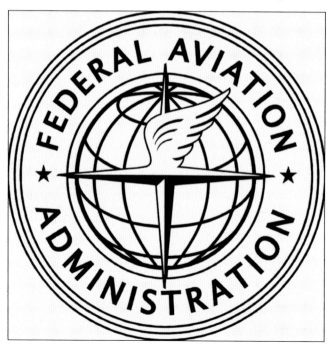

The Federal Aviation Agency, as part of the Department of Transportation, had jurisdiction over all aviation in the United States, including commercial and private operations. George Milligan, Mercy Flights' founder, was an employee of the FAA (as a control tower operator) but also an opponent of the FAA (as the chairman of the board of Mercy Flights). In addition to local concerns about Mercy Flights' sustainability, fledgling air ambulance companies throughout the United States had a strong interest in the impact of the Mercy Flights deliberations and subsequent FAA decisions.

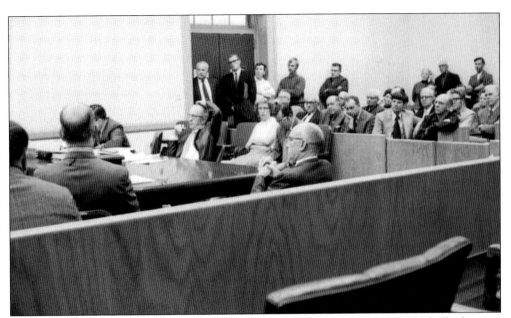

The FAA hearing began on October 20, 1971, at the federal courthouse in Medford. The hearing was well attended by the press and community leaders. In this picture, attorney Otto Frohnmayer (near the center, with his hand on his head) is shown along with Mercy Flights board member, secretary, and attorney Jeanette Marshall (seated behind Frohnmayer) and Mercy Flights founder George Milligan (in the center foreground with his face shown in profile). (Courtesy of the Southern Oregon Historical Society.)

SUMMARY: As an air taxi commercial operator, Mercy Flights would lose: all of its volunteer flight crews and ground help; all outright donations presently deductible; most subscriptions presently deductible; tax exempt status; free medical counseling with doctors on flight medical problems; gas tax rebate; low operating and maintenence costs; and the pilot perogatives allowed under Part 91 would be replaced by government controls exerted under Part 135.

IN SHORT: MERCY FLIGHTS WOULD FAIL IMMEDIATELY, AND THERE WOULD NO LONGER BE A FULL TIME AIR AMBULANCE SERVICE IN OREGON, OR ANYWHERE ELSE IN THE ENTIRE UNITED STATES.

Among the documents presented by Mercy Flights at the FAA hearing was this concise note that described why Mercy Flights (and other air ambulance services) would fail if it were required to abide by federal regulations for air taxi services.

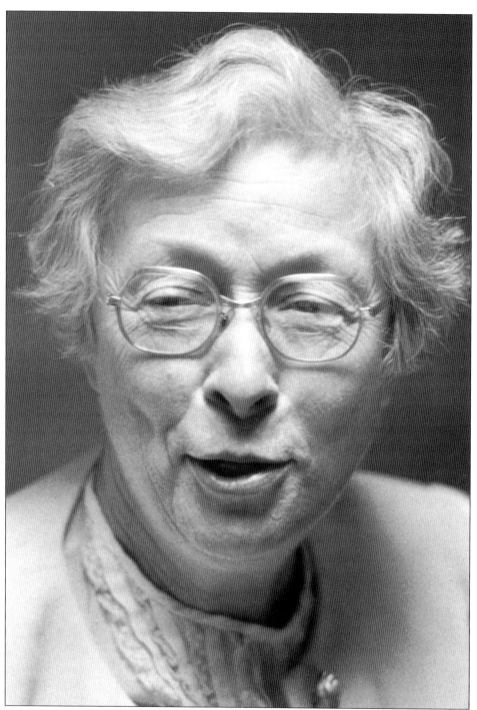

Medford attorney Jeanette Marshall served as secretary of the Mercy Flights board of directors from its inception and took meticulous records of board meetings and actions. She also united the Southern Oregon legal community, asking for help with specific topics as they arose. Marshall was key to persuading local attorney Otto Frohnmayer to represent Mercy Flights in their response to the actions taken by the Federal Aviation Agency. (Courtesy of the *Medford Mail Tribune*.)

SPECIAL MEETING OF THE BOARD
OF DIRECTORS OF MERCY FLIGHTS, INC.

June 19, 1972

A special meeting of the Board of Directors of Mercy Flights, Inc. was held at the airport manager's conference room at 10:00 o'clock A. M. on June 13, 1972. Directors present in person were George Milligan, George Flanagan, Dr. Jack Ingram, Eric Allen, Hazel Swayne, Jeannette Marshall, Gene Burrill, Henry Turk, Mike Burrill and Glen Jackson. Others present were F. A. A. Regional Director Chris Walk, Hearing Panel member and attorney Jonathan Howe, F. A. A. Chief, Flight Standards Bob Jones, also a panel member, and Bud Byerly, airport manager.

Mr. Walk stated that the purpose of the meeting was a friendly, informal discussion, that the F. A. A. was not trying to put Mercy Flights out of business, and that it was he who had asked for the "fact-finding" hearing. Several board members had copies of an F. A. A. "Briefing Package" or summary of tentative findings prepared after the hearing, and pointed out inaccuracies and distortions.

Jonathan Howe discussed his conclusions that Mercy Flights should be classed with the commercial operators to whom Part 135 is applicable because we charge money for transportation in our aircraft, and stated that it did not make any difference to him that Mercy Flights is a non-profit organization, indicating that they had others operating under Part 135 who didn't make any money either. Board members tried to point out to him that non-profit and unprofitable were two very different concepts, and that there was danger in board members opinions that the organization would lose its tax-exempt status, its community position as recipient of donations, and other very basic characteristics of our operation if we became an "air taxi";

The chairman extended an invitation to the visitors to fly with Mercy Flights to the coast on a personal inspection tour. The invitation was declined and the meeting adjourned at 11:45. The regional director stated that a decision in the case would be transmitted to George Milligan by telegram on Tuesday, June 27.

_____
Jeannette Marshall
Secretary

The next step in the conflict between Mercy Flights and the FAA was a meeting held on June 13, 1972, between FAA representatives and the Mercy Flights board. Jeanette Marshall's report of the disturbing meeting, including a description of the message delivered by regional administrator Jonathan Howe, is detailed in the minutes from a special meeting of the Mercy Flights board of directors held on June 19, 1972. Howe was not supportive of Mercy Flights not-for-profit status and felt that commercial air status was more appropriate.

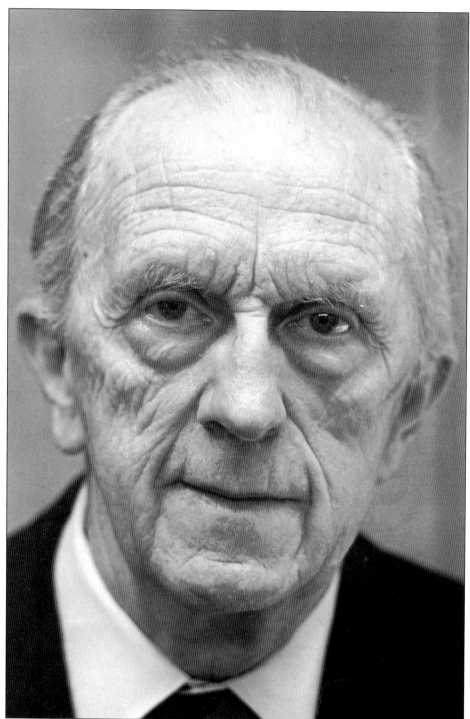

Medford attorney Otto Frohnmayer led the Mercy Flights legal and administrative team in their battle with the FAA regarding air ambulance rules. As the result of his efforts, and with the support of the Oregon congressional delegation, the FAA eventually reversed its original decision and developed specific rules for air ambulance operations. (Courtesy of the *Medford Mail Tribune*.)

OTTO J. FROHNMAYER
W. V. DEATHERAGE
STUART E. FOSTER
WILLIAM G. PURDY
DOUGLAS P. CUSHING

TELEPHONE
A/C 503 773-8425

June 26, 1972

Mr. Robert Whittington
Special Assistant to the
Administrator of Federal
Aviation Administration
Washington, D. C.

Re: Mercy Flights, Inc.

Dear Mr. Whittington:

As a result of the meeting held in Medford, Oregon between the
FAA and Mercy Flights on June 26, 1972, we felt it advisable to
set down on paper a possible solution to the problem. It was
apparent at the meeting that the effect of requiring Mercy Flights,
Inc. to apply for a certificate could have far-reaching legal effects
as follows:

      a. Its status as a nonprofit, charitable corporation.
      b. Its exemptions for gifts and bequests.
      c. Increased cost of operating, etc.

As a possible solution to the problem it is suggested that the
FARs be amended to recognize the existence of an air ambulance
operator as a separate classification.

This would eliminate the necessity of a finding that Mercy Flights,
Inc. is a commercial operator. The amendment would include the
broad classification of air ambulance operator within Part 135.
By amending the regulations in this manner, Mercy Flights would
be within the scope of Part 135, however, any possible adverse
effects of a finding that Mercy Flights is a commercial operator
would be avoided.

It is suggested that Part 135 be amended to include a special
section entitled "Air Ambulance Operations/Profit or Nonprofit".
This section would spell out in detail which of the portions of
Part 135 applied to the air ambulance operator and would also
delete certain portions of 135 which would not apply because of
the special nature of the operations.

Pending the amendment of Part 135 as suggested, Mercy Flights
would agree to comply with Part 135 with certain waivers to be
worked out between the Northwest Region and Mercy Flights,
however Mercy Flights cannot accept a certificate under Part 135
at this time.

In this June 26, 1972, letter to Robert Whittington, special assistant to the FAA administrator in Washington, DC, attorney Otto Frohnmayer suggested a solution to the Mercy Flights issue: the FAA should develop special regulations for air ambulances to allow them to best serve injured and ill patients throughout the United States.

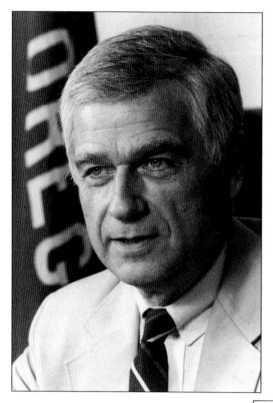

Willamette University president Mark Hatfield served as governor of Oregon from 1959 to 1967 and as a US senator from 1967 to 1997. Through the years, he and other members of the Oregon congressional delegation provided support to Mercy Flights as the FAA sought to place limits on Mercy Flights and other emerging air ambulance systems. On June 30, 1972, the FAA and Mercy Flights reached an agreement that would allow Mercy Flights to continue operating as a nonprofit air ambulance service. (Courtesy of the *Medford Mail Tribune*.)

The *Medford Mail Tribune* provided ongoing coverage of the Mercy Flights/FAA interactions. In this July 31, 1972, editorial, *Tribune* editor and Mercy Flights treasurer Eric Allen laid out the issues and called for ongoing community support. (Courtesy of the *Medford Mail Tribune*.)

4 A   Monday, July 31, 1972

MEDFORD MAIL TRIBUNE

An Independent Newspaper

Robert. W. Ruhl
(Publisher, 1919-1967; Editor, 1919-1958)

Mrs. Mabel W. Ruhi
Publisher

Eric W. Allen Jr.
Editor

Gerald T. Latham
General Manager

Earl H. Adams
Managing Editor

Mercy Flights and the FAA

Some day someone may decide to write a history of Mercy Flights, Inc., and if and when they do, one of the more interesting (and longer) chapters could be entitled "the FAA affair."

The FAA is the Federal Aviation Administration, part of the Department of Transportation, and it is charged with a lot of tasks, none of them easy, involving the regulation and safety of air traffic in the United States.

FOR YEARS, it has been puzzled by Mercy Flights, simply because it doesn't fit into any of the neat categories the FAA has set up for segments of the aviation industry. It isn't an airline, nor is it a private flying organization, nor is it an air taxi, nor is it a commercial organization.

It is, in fact, a non-profit, tax-exempt corporation, operated almost wholly with volunteer personnel, which provides air ambulance service in cases of medical need. It is not "for hire"; it flies only when a physician says his patient needs air transportation.

This is an old and familiar story to the people of southwestern Oregon, some thousands of whom help to support it through annual subscription fees, donations or bequests. But to the FAA, it was a puzzle, simply because there is nothing else like it anywhere in the world (except Lakeview, Ore., where another Mercy Flights, modeled after Medford's, has been in operation for a few years).

Since its first flight in January of 1950, Mercy Flights has been operating under Federal Aviation Regulations, Part 91, which pertains to private planes. For several years, the FAA has been worrying about this, and about two years ago it was decided that this category was inappropriate for an outfit that does transport people, and that makes a charge (when applicable) for the service.

So officers and directors of Mercy Flights received registered air mail letters to the effect that the organization would have to operate under Part 135, FAR, which governs air taxi-commercial flights, or face a "cease and desist" order.

In 1971 and 1972, the Federal Aviation Agency attempted to ground Mercy Flights because its lifesaving services did not adhere to federal air taxi regulations. A hearing in Medford, Oregon, followed by a ruling against Mercy Flights, led to public outcry. The intervention of Oregon's congressional delegation and a subsequent closer investigation of Mercy Flights' operation by Robert Whittington, special assistant to the FAA administrator, led to a reversal of the ruling. Whittington recommended that Mercy Flights be considered a model for similar services throughout the United States. Mercy Flights and its supporters celebrated with a festive dinner and awarded "Don't Call Us a Taxi" certificates to its many supporters.

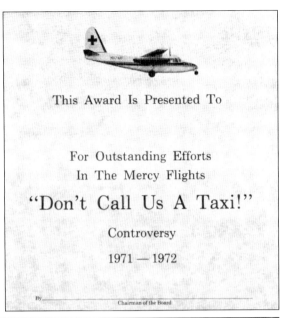

This Award Is Presented To

For Outstanding Efforts
In The Mercy Flights

"Don't Call Us A Taxi!"

Controversy

1971 — 1972

By_____
Chairman of the Board

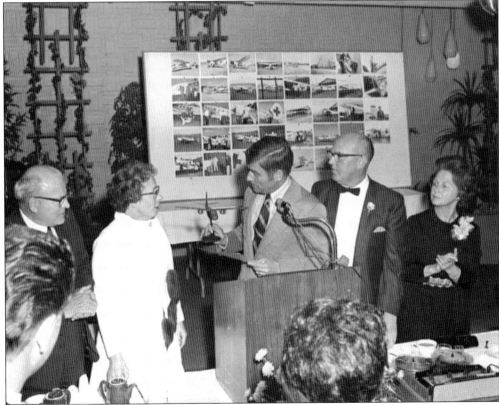

After the long—and ultimately successful—process with the FAA resulting in new federal rules for air ambulances, the community celebrated the outcome. Shown here with Sen. Mark Hatfield (at the podium) are, from left to right, Harry Marshall, Mercy Flights longtime board member and secretary Jeannette Marshall, Mercy Flights founder George Milligan, and Helene Milligan.

Mercy Flights wins new life

Mercy Flights Inc. of Medford this morning was spared expensive — and prohibitive — improvements when the Federal Aviation Administration withdrew air ambulance standards which it has been pushing for the past six years.

George Milligan, chairman of the board and chief pilot for the non-profit firm headquartered at the Medford-Jackson County Airport, said he learned of the action through the office of Sen. Bob Packwood, R-Ore.

"The standards would have stopped our service here as well as service everywhere else in the country," said Milligan. "There would've been no air ambulance service except for the very rich."

He said the standards would have forced Mercy Flights to buy new aircraft worth between $250,000 and $1 million apiece. Value of aircraft now in use ranges from $25,000 to $50,000.

"The point that we beat them on is that medical standards and licensing is a state prerogative," said Milligan. "Air and ground ambulance standards can be only what communities at the state level or the local level can afford."

Milligan said the standards would have required "all kinds of fancy things like hard hats and crowbars and snakebite kits."

Mercy Flights is supported by subscriber rates of $10 per year and by fees to non-subscribers who need emergency air service and live within the 400-mile radius service area.

For six years, the FAA pushed to establish air ambulance standards that included requirements for expensive planes and unnecessary infrastructure. Adherence to these standards would have put a halt to Mercy Flights' service. As described in the August 8, 1978, issue of the *Medford Mail Tribune*, these prohibitive policies were withdrawn. (Courtesy of the *Medford Mail Tribune*.)

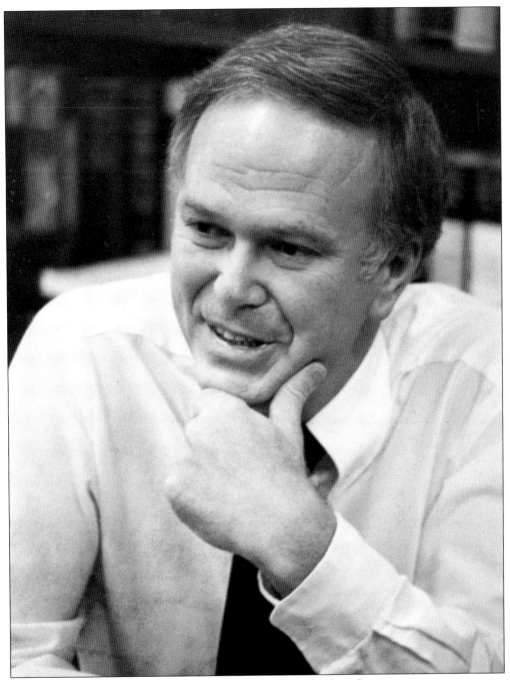

Sen. Bob Packwood, along with every other member of Congress from Oregon, was a strong supporter of Mercy Flights. They went through negotiations with the Federal Aviation Administration to create and update regulations to allow air ambulance services to exist and thrive in the often difficult environment of commercial aviation. Senator Packwood was the main Congressional opponent to the FAA's proposed regulations in 1978. (Courtesy of the *Medford Mail Tribune*.)

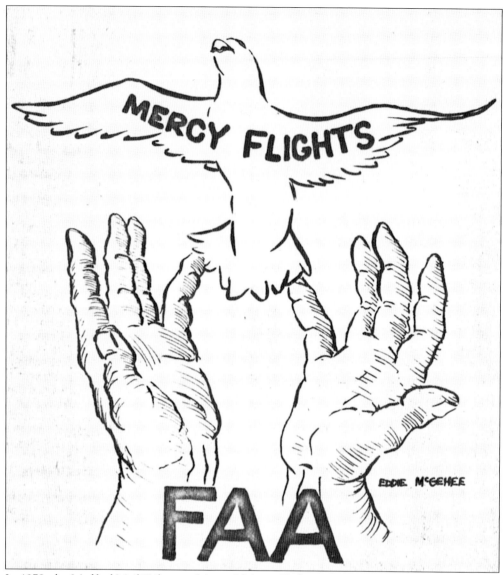

In 1978, the *Medford Mail Tribune* celebrated Mercy Flights' victory in its battle with the FAA with an editorial by Eric Allen and this illustration depicting the end result of Mercy Flights' interactions with the FAA. (Courtesy of *the Medford Mail Tribune*.)

Four

Challenges and Historic Rescues

Prior to 1983, when Emergency Medicine System legislation was passed in Oregon, rescues and emergency responses were informal. The idea of a "first responder" was a new concept. From the first days of its creation, Mercy Flights' history included involvement in precarious and dramatic rescues from unlikely landing strips such as sandbars and rural highways. Mercy Flights founder George Milligan often described these as "make-believe airports." In one of the early missions, a pilot and nurse landed in Agness, a small community on the Rogue River, and then had to hike to locate the injured patient.

Because of the outdoor lifestyle of rural Oregonians, rescues are commonplace in forests, rivers, lakes, on mountains, or even on sandbars. Fortunately, Mercy Flights' maneuverable single-engine planes, such as a Stinson Reliant or a Cessna 180, provided access to remote landing strips before helicopters became available. Milligan described the airstrip at Agness on the Rogue River as such: "It's a short strip. You get one chance. You either make it or you don't." Fortunately, Mercy Flights always made it.

Mercy Flights was also the first to respond to the 1955 Roseburg, Oregon, dynamite explosion that leveled the city; they immediately flew in utility workers and medical supplies. On more than one occasion, Mercy Flights delivered food and medications to small communities isolated by floods and forest fires. Several local pilots—who also volunteered for Mercy Flights—pioneered early fog-dispersal technology that was later used by Mercy Flights and United Airlines to allow planes to land at the Medford Airport through breaks in the dense freezing fog. Mercy Flights also routinely flew federal officials on missions to photograph and assess flood and fire damage. After 1983, when Emergency Medical Systems were created, Mercy Flights' interventions were less immediately needed in disasters and emergencies, but they remained active in support of the EMS responses and initiatives.

Despite his full-time job as an FAA control tower operator, Milligan led and managed Mercy Flights and was a constant presence at the Medford Airport. His personal leadership through rescues, first responses, and disasters was recognized by a number of state and national aviation and safety agencies.

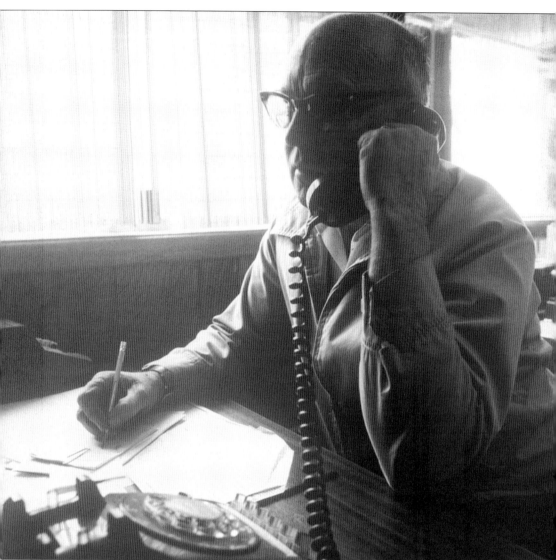

In a time when telephones were the only method of communication, Mercy Flights' staff and pilots were in constant phone contact about their locations and availability. Founder George Milligan pioneered the use of radios and some of the first beepers to increase the speed of Mercy Flights' rapid responses to medical emergencies.

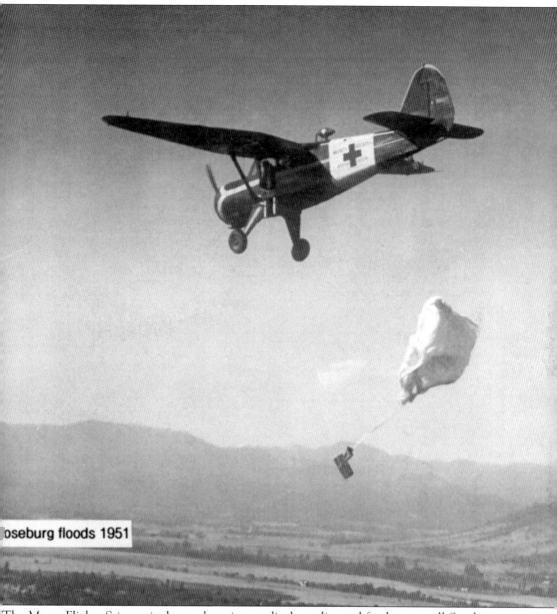

oseburg floods 1951

The Mercy Flights Stinson is shown dropping medical supplies and food to a small Southern Oregon community isolated by floods. Without a formal emergency system in place for the entire state of Oregon until 1983, Mercy Flights was most often the first to appear when small communities—even those without an airstrip—needed help.

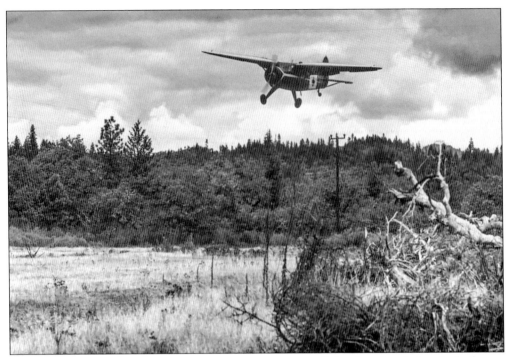

Early airstrips in small and remote communities were not well developed and often looked more like pastures. In some small towns, such as Happy Camp, California, the main street of the town was cleared to serve as a landing strip, with the headlights of gathered automobiles illuminating the area and guiding the pilot into the small space. In this photograph, a Mercy Flights Stinson Reliant is landing at a remote field in the Oregon Cascade Mountains.

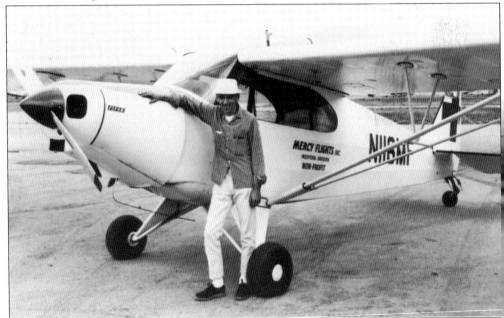

Early Mercy Flights pilot Bill Florey is shown with the second Mercy Flights single-engine plane, a Piper Cub. (Courtesy of the Southern Oregon Historical Society.)

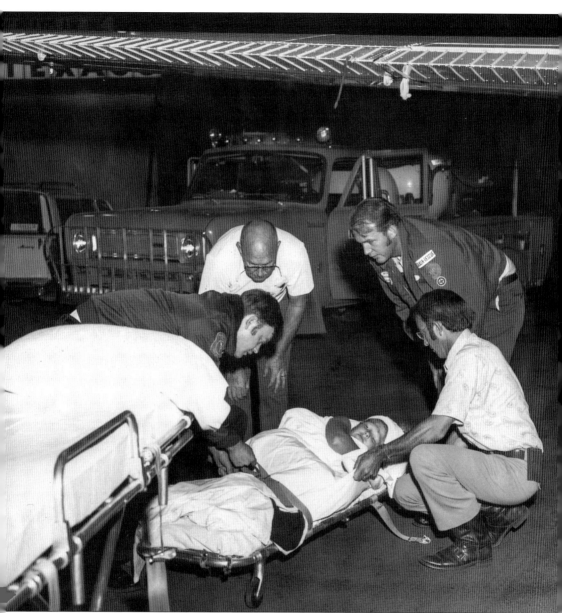

Even before helicopters were in use, Mercy Flights transferred injured patients from remote locations. Here, two unidentified firefighters, along with George Milligan (center, in the white shirt) and Jackson County sheriff Duane Franklin (crouching at right; also a Mercy Flights pilot), are shown under a Mercy Flights plane wing as they are loading a patient for transfer to a regional medical center.

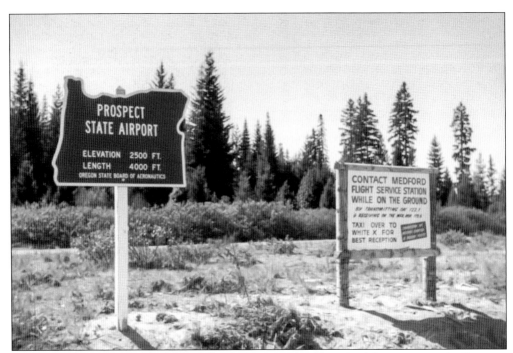

An official State of Oregon sign describes the elevation and length of the runway at the Prospect State Airport, which was located in a small lumbering community north of Medford en route to Crater Lake.

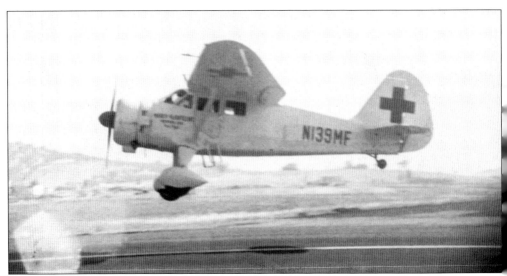

Mercy Flights' Stinson is shown landing at a rural and remote airstrip in the course of a rescue.

Lumberman Eugene F. Burrill and his wife, Gladys, lived in the small community of Prospect, Oregon, outside of Medford; they were strong supporters of Mercy Flights. As pilots themselves, they supported the expansion of aviation in Southern Oregon as well as Mercy Flights endeavors. (Courtesy of the *Medford Mail Tribune*.)

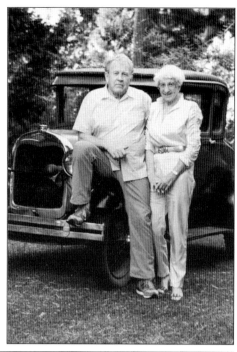

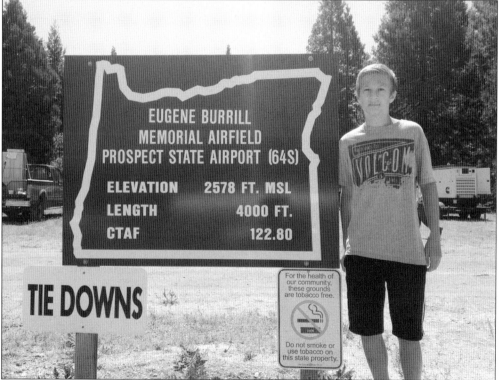

In honor of his contributions to the Prospect flying community, the strip at the Prospect State Airport was renamed Eugene Burrill Memorial Airfield. Eugene and Gladys' great-grandson Parker Burrill is shown standing next to the memorial sign. (Courtesy of Michael E. Burrill Jr.)

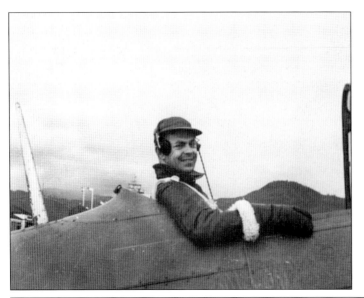

Gene Kooser was one of Mercy Flights' first pilots. A World War II pilot, Kooser and his business partner, Harvey Brandau, pioneered fog-seeding techniques at the Medford Airport; these were later used by both United Airlines and Mercy Flights to facilitate landings by dispersing and clearing freezing fog above the Medford runway. (Courtesy of the Southern Oregon Historical Society.)

Medford, Home Of Fog-Seeding,

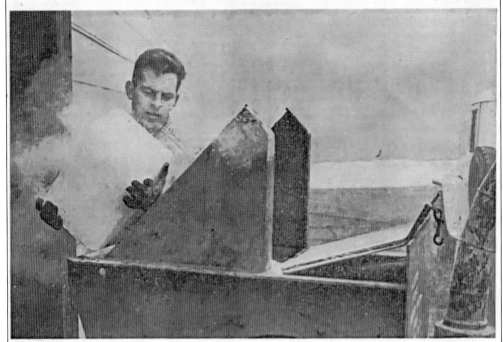

DENNIS CONNER, PILOT of fog-seeding plane, dumps block of dry ice into chipper which shreds it into flakes. Some 415 pounds was dumped into fog over Medford's airport in 65 minutes last Saturday before swath was cleared sufficient for two United airliners to land, take-off. Air was too warm—34 degrees—for best results.

The Medford Airport is often weathered in during winter storms and freezing fog, which make it impossible for pilots to land. Two Mercy Flights pilots, Harvey Brandau and Gene Kooser, pioneered a dry-ice fog-seeding operation that was later adopted by Mercy Flights to clear the fog directly above the runway. This image and the two on the following page are clippings from an article that appeared in the *News-Review* in Roseburg, Oregon, in December 1951.

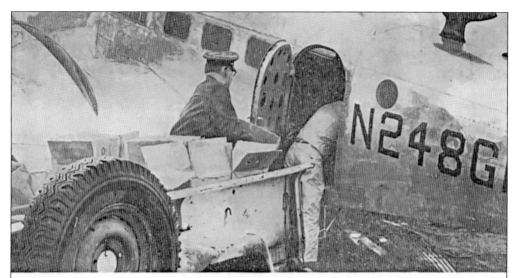

TWIN-ENGINED Beechcraft of Aero-Ag, above, was loaded with boxes of dry ice by Bowker and Mortimer for experimental seeding. Harvey Brandau and Eugene Kooser of Medford were first to prove success of dry ice in clearing fog. George Milligan, Wings of Mercy president, Medford, has been seeding fog for ten years.

A small plane could still take off with limited visibility, drop dry ice crystals to super-cool the fog (causing it to dissipate), and then land on the runway. The City of Medford contracted with local operators, such as Aero-Ag and Mercy Flights, for fog seeding so that bigger planes from United Airlines could access the airport. This process, which now uses helium balloons, is still being refined at the Rogue Valley International–Medford Airport.

Performs 'Miracle' For Camera

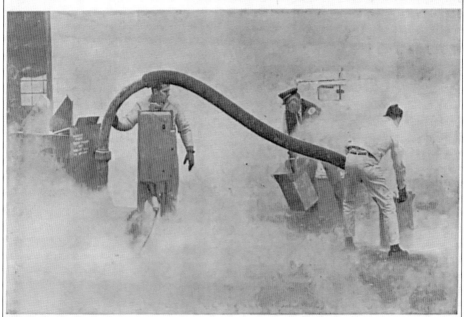

DRY ICE "SEED" is boxed with aid of Charles Mortimer, of United (in cap) and Jay Bowker, Conner's copilot. Airport runway remained clear for hour and half after seeding, while fog blanketed rest of valley. Conner and Bowker of Aero-Ag Co., have contract with city of Medford to clear away fog when required.

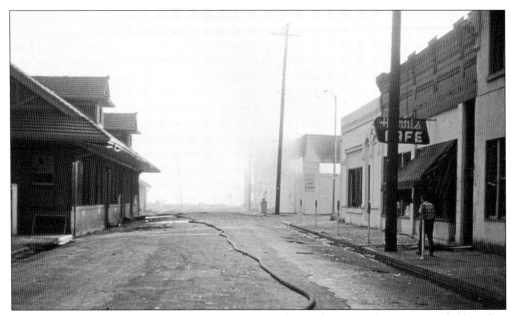

On August 7, 1959, Mercy Flights was a first responder to the tragic dynamite truck blast that leveled downtown Roseburg, Oregon. A fire in a nearby building ignited a dynamite truck that was illegally parked and carrying a two-ton load of dynamite and four-and-one-half tons of ammonium nitrate. The blast leveled eight city blocks, killed 14 people, and injured many others. This photograph illustrates the type of devastation that was experienced by the locals. (Courtesy of the Douglas County Historical Society)

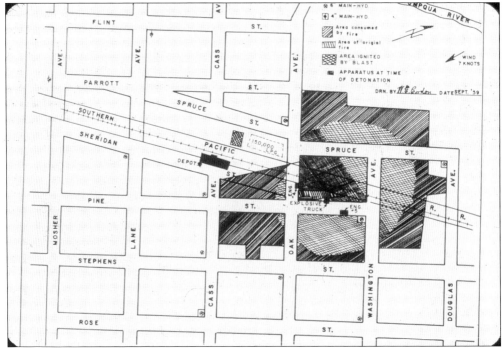

A map of downtown Roseburg, Oregon, shows the location and pattern of damage of the Roseburg dynamite blast on August 7, 1959. (Courtesy of the Douglas County Historical Society.)

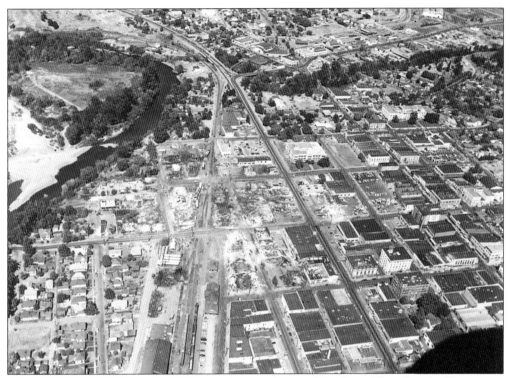

The large scale of the damage is evident in this aerial view of Roseburg. Three hundred businesses within a 30-block radius were damaged by the blast. Of those, 72 were declared structurally unsafe, requiring major repairs and renovation. Twelve buildings beyond the eight-block perimeter were condemned. The face of Roseburg changed forever in an instant. The explosion became commonly known to locals as "the Blast." (Courtesy of the Douglas County Historical Society.)

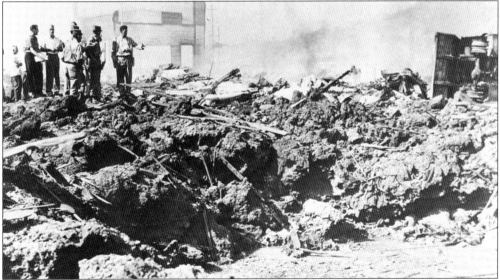

Fortunately, many lives were spared by that fact that the Roseburg blast took place in the middle of the night, when downtown Roseburg was essentially unoccupied. The crater created by the blast was 22 feet in diameter and 12 feet deep. (Courtesy of the Douglas County Historical Society.)

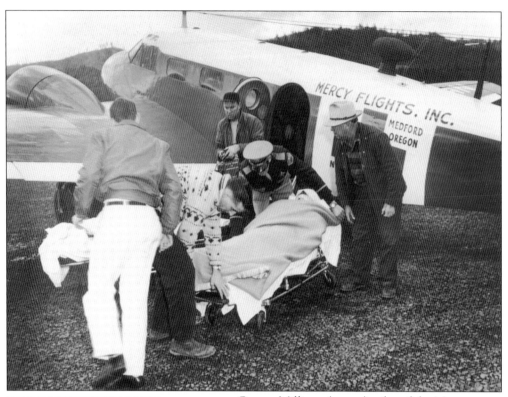

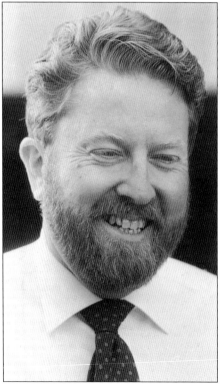

George Milligan (center), pilot of the Mercy Flights Twin Beechcraft, is shown overseeing the loading of an unidentified patient at a remote airstrip with the assistance of a local police officer and copilot Fred Hale (far right). Prior to federal support of local emergency medical services in the late 1970s and early 1980s, many ambulance crews had little medical training and simply existed to transport patients to the nearest appropriate resources.

As a pilot and longtime board member, Michael E. Burrill Sr. led Mercy Flights through some of its biggest challenges. Described by the *Medford Mail Tribune* as "a longtime industrialist, developer and community supporter," he received the First Citizen Award from the Medford Chamber of Commerce in 2009. In addition to his Mercy Flights leadership, Burrill has served on a variety of boards, including the Oregon State Aviation Board and Oregon State Board of Forestry, as well as those of the Oregon Community Foundation, Southern Oregon University Foundation, Southern Oregon Regional Economic Development Inc., and Oregon State Criminal Justice Commission. (Courtesy of the *Medford Mail Tribune*.)

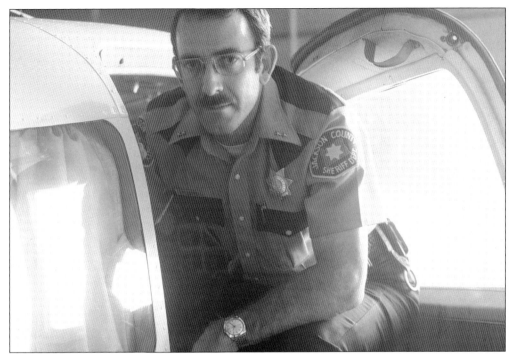

Medford sheriff Duane Franklin, a former Oregon state policeman, was also a Mercy Flights pilot and expert on difficult rescues.

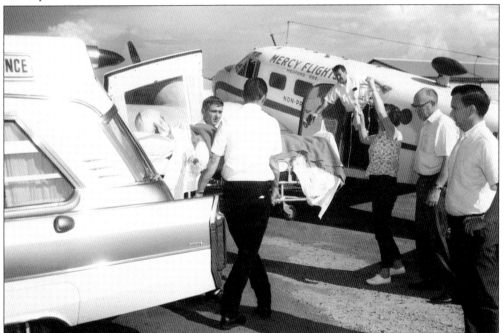

In June 1969, Chester Adams, manager of the American Propane Company, was severely burned in a propane truck. Mercy Flights flew him from Rogue Valley Hospital to San Francisco. The *Medford Mail Tribune* reported that the stretcher from the Mercy Flights plane was used by the ambulance service attendants to reduce the number of moves for the patient.

"THIS IS THE TOWER. SAY AGAIN?"

Air Traffic Controllers hear many heart-stopping announcements over their radios, but during 28 years in the business, I'd never heard one equal to the impact which brought everything to a halt in the FAA Control Tower, at Medford, Oregon, Dec. 5, 1969.

As they might say on Dragnet, "It was murky in Medford. I was working the day watch in the glass house. My partners were Baker, Brinkman, and Seeberger." The ceiling was 700 feet overcast, with visibility about a mile and a half, in light snow and fog. Two thousand feet above, the fog ended in bright blue sky, and you could see a hundred miles, if you were fortunate or unfortunate enough to be there, depending of course on your airman's qualifications, and your aircraft.

One of those in the unfortunate category was a man whom we'd been talking to for about five minutes, and who needed to land shortly, because his aircraft was low on fuel. Simple enough, as there was a nice airport, fog-free, up towards Crater Lake, and only about thirty miles away, at Prospect, Oregon.

Our difficulty with the "fuel-needer" was that he didn't seem to be able to take directions, or understand the information that we needed, like altitude, aircraft heading, and fuel remaining. He brought everything to a stop with his coup de grace: "I know nothing about airplanes. This is not the pilot. The pilot is a deaf mute!".

In addition to flying, George Milligan enjoyed writing. Here, he tells the story of a distress call from a small plane over Medford that was running out of fuel and could not find the airport through the thick clouds; this was made all the more challenging by the fact the pilot was deaf and mute. Unable to radio instructions to the pilot, Milligan took to the air in Iron Annie to lead the plane to a safe landing in Prospect.

Mercy Flights pilot Don Wilson took part in many Mercy Flights missions and rescues over the years.

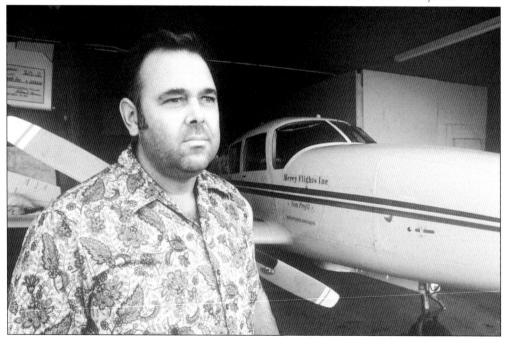

76

Five

ESTABLISHING SOUTHERN OREGON AS A REGIONAL MEDICAL CENTER

As the population of Southern Oregon increased, so did the need for health care at all levels. In the 1940s and 1950s, small community hospitals in the region offered the most basic emergency, medical, surgical, and obstetrical services. Mercy Flights became the region's solution for rapidly transferring complex patients to Level 1 and Level 2 hospitals in urban centers in Portland (263 road miles away) and San Francisco (373 road miles away).

In the 1960s, Medford's two community hospitals grew into more complex health-care systems that offered care across all of the medical and surgical specialties and subspecialties. Sacred Heart Hospital, part of the Providence healthcare system, built a new facility and renamed it Providence Hospital. The Medford Community Hospital also built a new facility and renamed it Rogue Valley Memorial Hospital. With these new campuses that included contiguous medical offices, treatment centers, rehabilitation facilities, and laboratory services, Medford was now on the map as a regional medical center located midway between Portland and San Francisco.

While some patients were still transferred to Portland and San Francisco, the balance of Mercy Flights' services shifted to transfers from small hospitals and clinics in rural and often remote communities to Medford. New technologies also played a major role, as Mercy Flights began to provide neonatal transfer services for premature and ill infants as well as more complex inflight monitoring in pressurized aircraft for very ill patients.

New technology also brought with it the need for more highly trained crews, including paramedics and specialty care nurses. Medical and nursing advisors to Mercy Flights provided recommendations and monitoring for these complex new services.

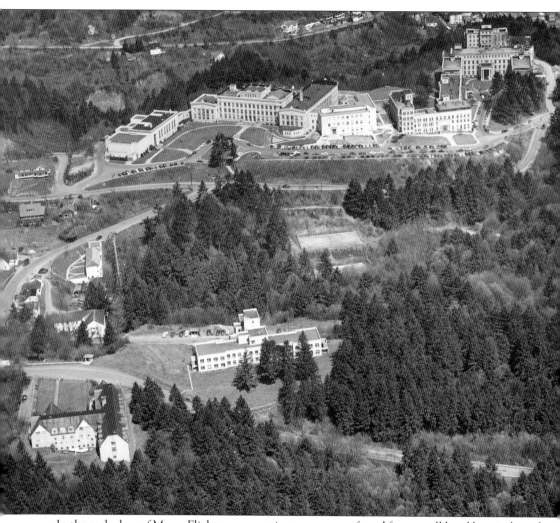

In the early days of Mercy Flights, many patients were transferred from small local hospitals to the University Hospital in Portland, Oregon, where a full range of specialties were available. Shown in this 1950 photograph is the hospital complex in Portland, which included a VA hospital and the Shriners' children's hospital. Upon landing in Portland, patients still had to endure an ambulance ride through busy urban traffic before making slow progress up the winding road to the hospital on the hill. (Courtesy of OHSU Historical Collections & Archives.)

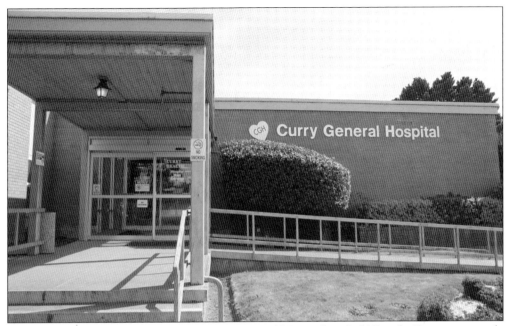

Rural coastal hospitals—such as the Curry General Hospital in Gold Beach, Oregon—provide basic services in what are now called Critical Access Hospitals. In the 1950s, part of their job was to stabilize patients and arrange for their quick transfer by air, which enabled them to avoid long ground trips on treacherous two-lane rural highways.

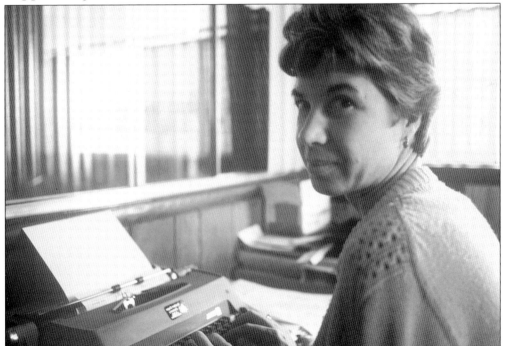

Diane Coash was Mercy Flights' manager and carried out many tasks, including dispatching flights, coordinating crews, managing supplies, and even personally typing out each individual Mercy Flights membership card, which were replaced annually.

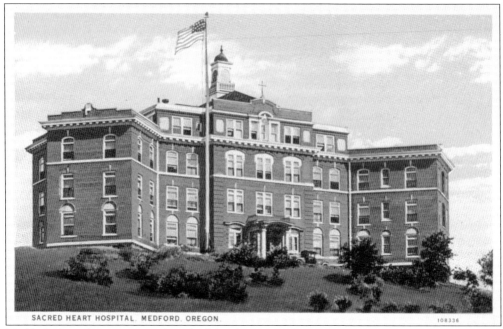

SACRED HEART HOSPITAL. MEDFORD. OREGON.

Medford's Sacred Heart Hospital was built by the Sisters of Providence at the request of a committee of physicians, who petitioned the organization to found a hospital in the growing town of Medford in 1910. Dedicated in 1912, the hospital was located on the highest hill in East Medford and soon opened a nursing school. Early graduate Hazel Swayne served as Mercy Flights' chief nurse for many years. (Courtesy of Providence Archives.)

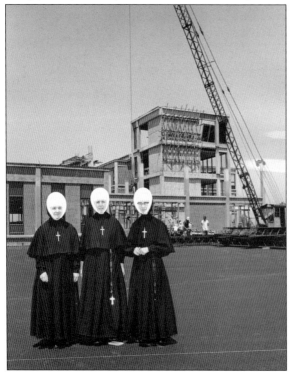

Administrative and nursing leaders from the Sisters of Providence supervised the building of the new Providence Hospital on Crater Lake Avenue in Medford, which was dedicated in 1966. The name of Medford's original Catholic hospital, Sacred Heart, was changed to Providence Hospital in keeping with other name changes within the regional Providence system. (Courtesy of Providence Archives.)

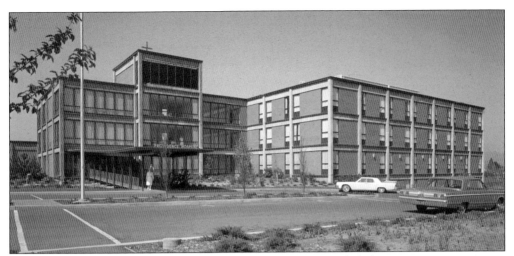

State of the art when it opened in 1966, Providence Hospital included 93 private patient rooms. The hospital was also equipped with the most modern equipment to provide a broader range of services and specialties. (Courtesy of Providence Archives.)

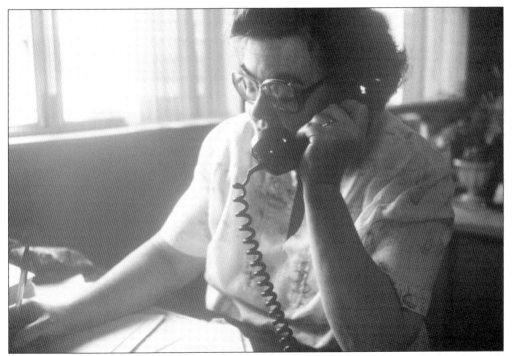

Medical staff in Mercy Flights' coverage area had 24-hour access to Mercy Flights dispatch services. Here, Dorothy Park, a Mercy Flights staff member, is shown in conversation with a hospital emergency room.

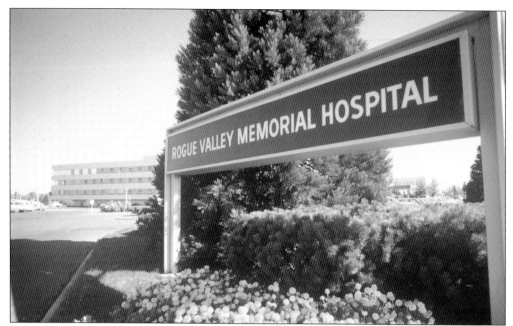

The small Medford Community Hospital, located on Medford's Main Street, was expanded and rebuilt as Rogue Valley Memorial Hospital in 1956. Rogue Valley, along with Providence hospitals, serve the Southern Oregon/Northern California region. Originally small community hospitals, Rogue Regional Medical Center and Providence-Medford Medical Center can now provide the highest levels of care across all specialties, reversing Mercy Flights patterns of transporting patients to Portland and bringing all levels of care for the Southern Oregon region into Medford.

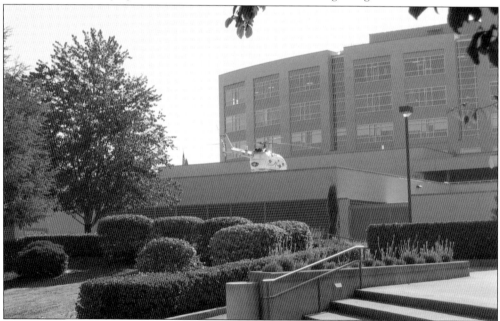

In December 2012, this hospital was renamed Rogue Regional Memorial Center and is now part of the Asante Health System. It continues to expand to support the needs of residents of the Southern Oregon region.

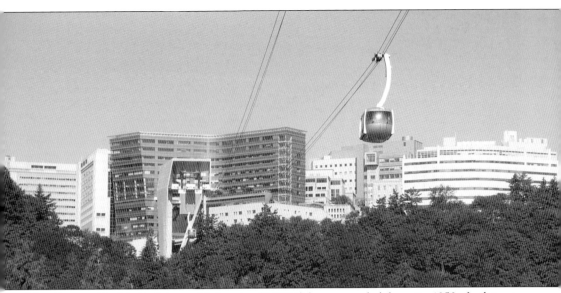

The Oregon Health & Science University (OHSU) has expanded from its 1950s facilities to include new buildings along the Willamette River that are accessible from the hill by an aerial tram systems and include a new veterans' hospital, a new Shriners' hospital, and an expanded university hospital. (Courtesy of OHSU Historical Collections & Archives.)

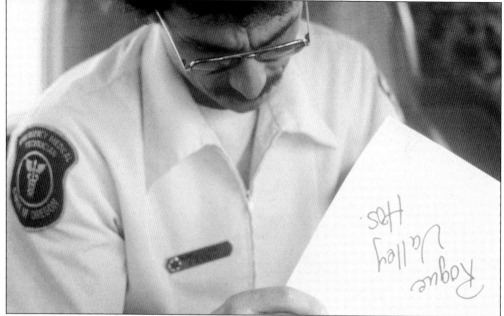

Governmental Emergency Medical Services were developed in the early 1970s and included the development and utilization of paramedics and EMTs as well as advanced monitoring and communication systems used during patient transports. Here, a local paramedic is reviewing a patient's chart for transfer to Rogue Valley Memorial Hospital.

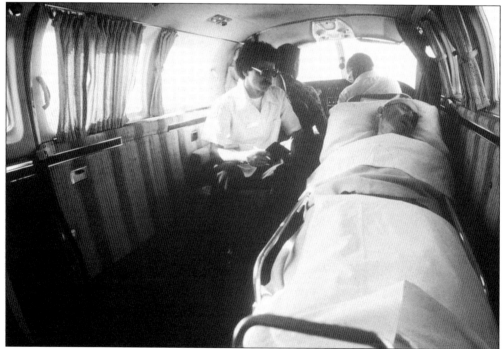

Over time, Mercy Flights acquired larger and faster planes that were also more comfortable for patients, nurses, paramedics, and pilots. Here, Mercy Flights crew members are shown with a patient as they prepare for a departure to more complex medical facilities in Portland, Oregon.

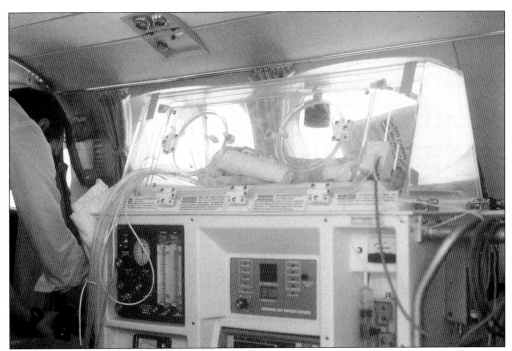

As incubators and the new medical specialty of neonatology developed, premature infants miraculously survived their early births. In 1986, the American Academy of Pediatrics published *Guidelines for Air and Ground Transportation of Pediatric Patients.* Mercy Flights actively worked with hospitals to provide this important transport, which also involved specially trained nurses and respiratory therapists. Medford's Rogue Valley Memorial Hospital received and cared for premature infants from throughout Southern Oregon and Northern California. A neonatal transport unit is pictured here inside a Mercy Flights air ambulance.

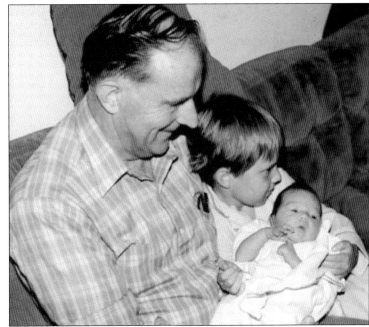

Medford pediatrician Dr. Hank Boehnke, who was also a pilot and Mercy Flights advisor on neonatal transport, is pictured with his grandson Jacob and his infant granddaughter Emily. (Courtesy of Joan Smith.)

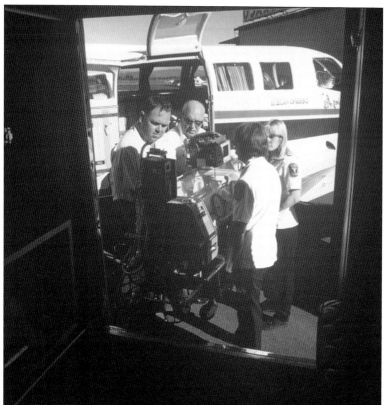

Over time, the intense neonatal transports became even more complex, requiring additional space in the Mercy Flights planes. Here, Don Wilson (at far left) and George Milligan (next to Wilson) are shown with a Mercy Flights crew during the first steps of a neonatal transport.

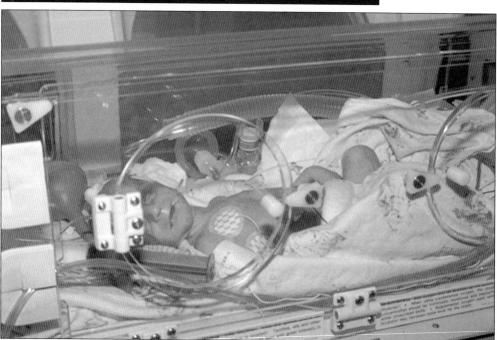

This close-up of an infant in a neonatal transport unit provides a glimpse of the small size and vulnerability of these very special patients.

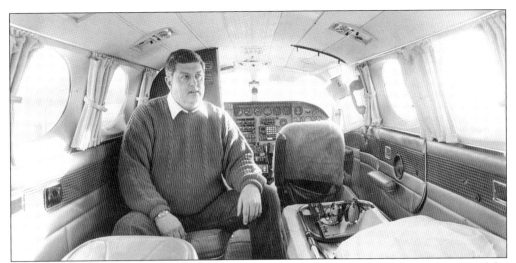

Ron Tycer, appointed general manager of Mercy Flights in January 1992, is pictured in one of the organization's then-newest planes around the time of his appointment. (Courtesy of the *Medford Mail Tribune*.)

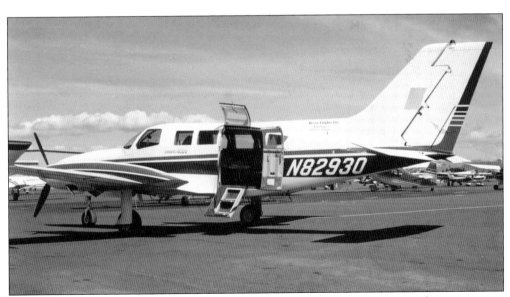

Newer planes still required modifications, particularly to the doors, to accommodate patients on stretchers. Each modification and adaptation was submitted to the FAA for approval.

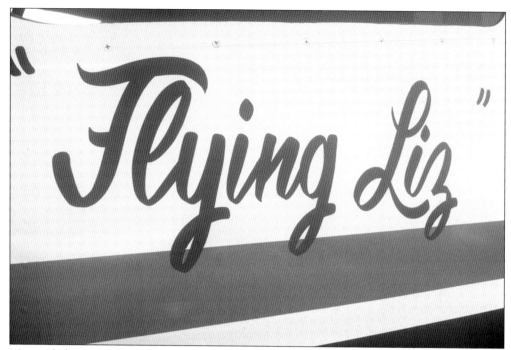

Mercy Flights purchased Flying Liz, a Cessna 402B, in May 1980 with the support of *Medford Mail Tribune* editor and Mercy Flights board member Eric Allen and his wife, Liz. She was later transported, via Mercy Flights, back and forth to Portland for treatment a number of times.

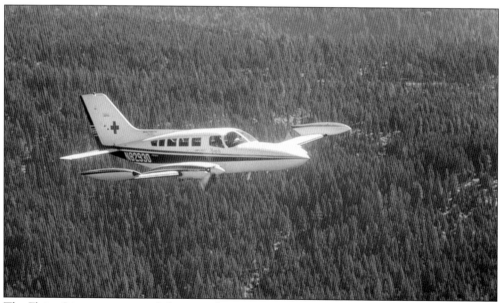

The Flying Liz was pressurized, faster, and more comfortable for patients who required complex care while in the transport.

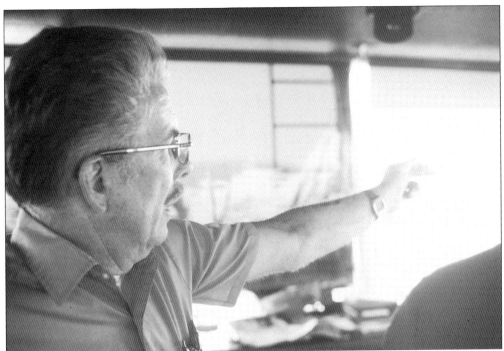

The support base for Mercy Flights at the Medford Airport included a wide range of individuals, including the FAA control tower operators at the Medford Control Tower. Some of the control operators, like George Milligan, were also Mercy Flights pilots. Jack Buckley is pictured here at work in the Medford Tower.

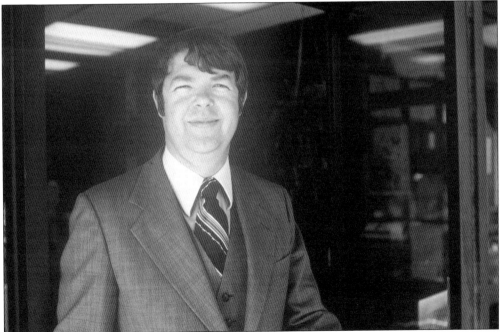

Ron Fields served as Medford Airport manager from 1972 to 1978 and presided over the rapid growth and development of the airport.

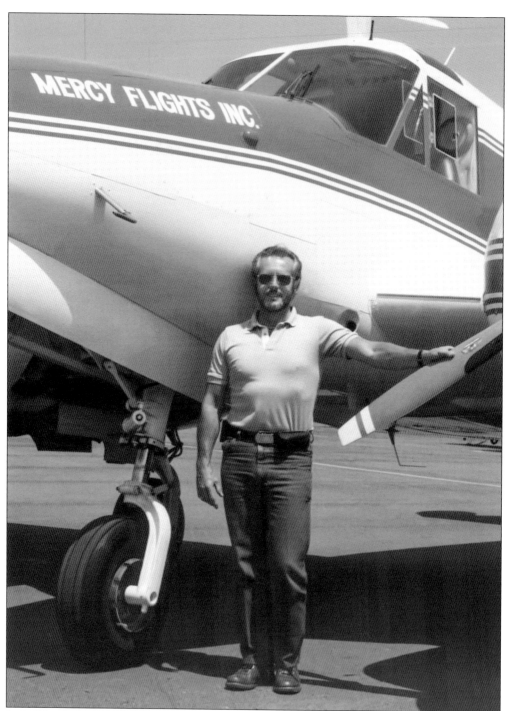

Jack Wheeler, Mercy Flights pilot and FAA control tower operator, is pictured at Mercy Flights' headquarters. A former military pilot, Wheeler worked closely with pilots and paramedics as new technology, such as neonatal transport, was integrated into Mercy Flights. Wheeler also informally served as the Mercy Flights historian and collected and preserved photographs and memorabilia related to Mercy Flights.

Six

RESPONSE TO TRAGEDY

While Mercy Flights grew and expanded in the 1980s, this was also the darkest time for the air ambulance service. On February 9, 1985, an icy Saturday morning, Mercy Flights twin-engine Aero Commander unexpectedly lost power, crashed, and exploded in a field less than a mile from the Medford–Jackson County Airport.

The crew included Mercy Flights founder George Milligan, beloved Medford pediatrician Dr. Henry Boehnke, and Mercy Flights paramedic Steve Trosin. The elderly patient was being transferred to Medford from Gold Beach. Copilot Boehnke was a volunteer pilot for Mercy Flights and served on its board of directors. He had logged more than 1,100 hours and also had a commercial pilot's license as well as instrument and multi-engine aircraft ratings.

According to United Press International (UPI), "The pilot of an air ambulance plane that crashed on a medical mission guided his aircraft away from a populated area before it crashed and exploded . . . killing all four aboard, witnesses said."

Upon news of the crash, the Mercy Flights board immediately met to assess the tragedy and to assure the community of Mercy Flights' safety record and the stability of the organization.

The FAA's investigation of the crash was fraught with controversy and conflict about the cause of the crash. Residents of the region wrote and spoke about their own personal experiences with Mercy Flights' history of saving lives and supported ongoing service.

In 1989, a second crash—Mercy Flights' turboprop Beechcraft King Air crashed while attempting to land in the fog at Gold Beach Airport— resulted in the loss of three Mercy Flights crew members: pilot Richard Mendolia, copilot Wally Nitowski, and flight nurse Diane Lefler.

In response to each of these tragedies, there was an outpouring of support from friends, patients, doctors, and community leaders blessing the heroic Mercy Flights crew members and acknowledging their contributions to the communities served by Mercy Flights.

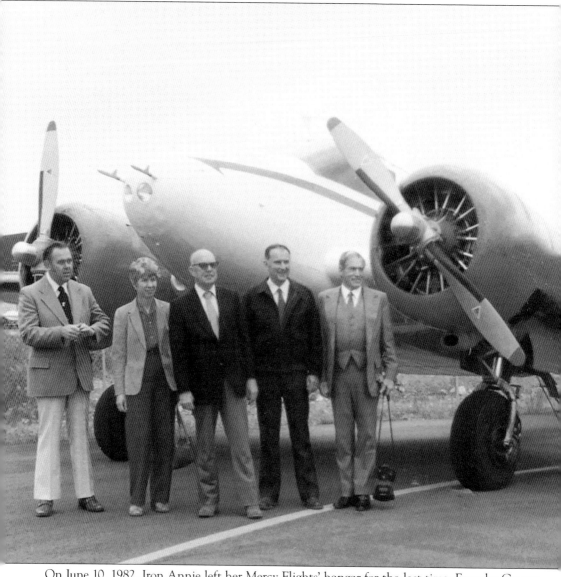

On June 10, 1982, Iron Annie left her Mercy Flights' hangar for the last time. Founder George Milligan (center), accompanied by, from left to right, Don Wilson, Diane Coash, Dr. Hank Boehnke, and Cliff Cheney, took the plane to Boeing Field in Seattle to turn her over to the Museum of Flight.

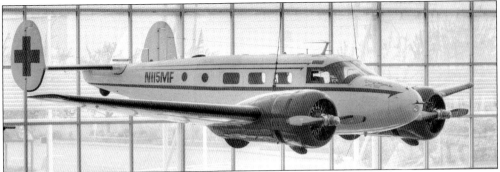

During 21 years of service with Mercy Flights, the plane known as Iron Annie had carried 1,150 patients. Eugene F. Burrill Lumber Company bought Iron Annie to donate to the Museum of Flight, where she now hangs on display at the south end of the building. (Courtesy of Geoff Collins.)

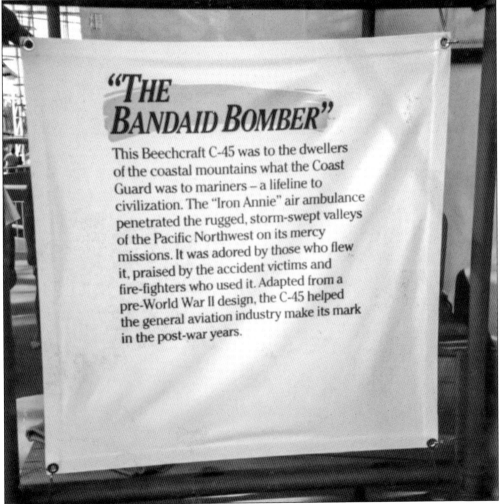

This placard for the "Band-Aid [sic] Bomber" (also known as Iron Annie) describes the unique rescue capabilities and experiences of the Twin Beechcraft and her responses to emergencies in rural southwestern Oregon.

93

Mercy flight crashes; 4 die

MEDFORD (AP) — Four people, including the founder of the nation's only non-profit volunteer air ambulance service, were killed Saturday when an ambulance plane crashed and burst into flames near the Medford-Jackson County airport, authorities said.

George E. Milligan, 65, the founder of Mercy Flights Inc., was the plane's pilot, said Donald E. Wilson, Mercy Flights' chief operations officer.

The other victims were two crew members and a patient. Wilson identified them as Dr. Henry Boehnke, the plane's co-pilot; Steven Trosin, a paramedic; and patient Marjorie Olney, 71, of Brookings.

Boehnke was a Medford pediatrician. Trosin, also of Medford, was a paramedic who was volunteering his services for Saturday's flight, Wilson said.

Olney was being flown from

Curry General Hospital in Gold Beach on the Oregon Coast to Rogue Valley Medical Center in Medford, said Jeff Maldonado, chief deputy for the Jackson County Sheriff's Department.

The twin-engine Rockwell Aero Commander lost power as it approached the airport's north runway at 12:48 p.m., said Mike O'Connor, regional duty officer for the Federal Aviation Administration in Seattle.

"He was on an approach and

downwind from the runway when both his engines quit," O'Connor said. "Apparently, according to the tower, he made a left turn and went nose-down . . . into the ground."

The plane crashed near some houses in a cow pasture about a mile short of the runway. "They believe it exploded on impact," O'Connor said.

None of the debris struck the houses, said Cheryl Williams, a records clerk in the sheriff's office.

In his communication with the flight control tower at the airport, the pilot did not say what caused the plane's engine to quit, O'Connor said.

There was nothing unusual about the weather, and the pilot had followed normal procedures, he said.

FAA investigators from Portland and Seattle and a National Transportation Safety Board inspector

Turn to CRASH, Back Page.

On February 9, 1985, a Mercy Flights plane transporting an elderly patient from Gold Beach on the Oregon Coast crashed just north of the Medford Airport. Piloted by Mercy Flights founder George Milligan, with well-known Medford pediatrician Dr. Hank Boehnke serving as copilot, the flight also carried Mercy Flights' paramedic Steve Trosin. There were no survivors.

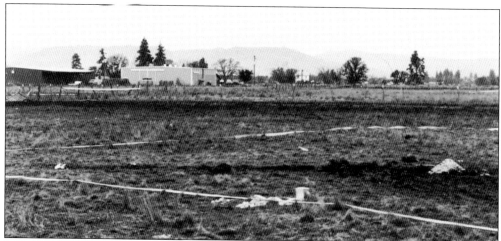

This photograph shows the scene of the Mercy Flights crash that occurred on February 9, 1985. The fiery crash resulted in the complete destruction of the aircraft, making it difficult to determine the cause of the accident.

Aircraft Number ___233W___   Round Trip Mileage ___160___

Date ___2-9-85___   Rate: __subscriber - 25%__

Patient Number ___7,369___   Fee: __n/c__

Mercy Flights, Inc.
PILOT'S FLIGHT REPORT

Flying Time:

Flight not completed due to
loss of aircraft, crew and
patient. God Bless You All.

Name of Patient: __Marjorie B. Olney__   Age: ___71___

Address: ███████████████████ Phone: _____

Employer: __retired__   Phone: _____

Address: _____

Bill To: __friend-Frank Akin__ ████████ _____

Address: _____

Nature of Emergency: __rule out polynephritis-possibly__

__colistitus.__   __Monitor-IV-oxygen__

Instructions: _____

Time of Request: __10:00am__   Depart MFR __11:00am__

Departure: ___CH___   Hospital ___Curry Gen'l___

Time of Take-off: _____   Physician ___Williams___

Destination: __Mfr__   Hospital ___RVMC___

Time of Arrival: _____   Physician ___Calloway___

Nurse: ___20.00___   Name: ___Steve Trosin___

Pilot: ___20.00___   Name: ___George E. Milligan___

Co-Pilot: ___10.00___   Name: ___Hank Boehnke___

Flight Authorized by: ___g em___

The flight report, submitted by Diane Coash in place of the pilot, reads: "Flight not completed due to loss of aircraft, crew and patient. God Bless You All."

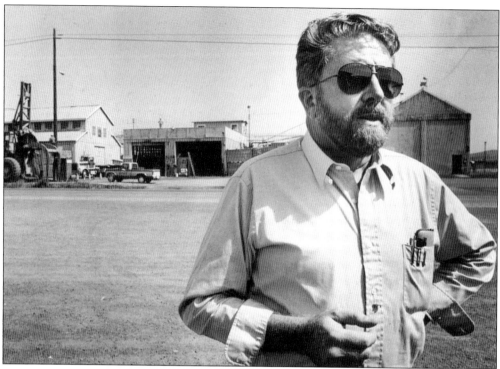

Since George Milligan was acting as both chairman of the board and general manager of Mercy Flights, his death left the organization without a definite leader. Longtime board member and fellow pilot Michael E. Burrill Sr. was closely involved in keeping Mercy Flights running immediately following the crash. (Courtesy of the *Medford Mail Tribune*.)

Tuesday, Feb. 12, 1985

Obituaries

Milligan service Thursday

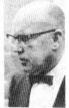

The memorial service for George E. Milligan, 65, of Jacksonville, who died Saturday, will be at 11 a.m. Thursday at the First Church of the Nazarene, 1974 E. McAndrews Road, Medford, with the Rev. Fred Milligan

Strasburg officiating. Memory Gardens Funeral Directors are in charge of arrangements.

Memorial contributions may be made to Mercy Flights Inc., P.O. Box 522, Medford.

Mr. Milligan was born Nov. 16, 1919, in St. Joseph, Mo. On Dec. 1, 1960, in Medford, he married the former Helene C. Prentice, who survives.

During World War II, Mr. Milligan served with the U.S. Army Air Corps as a radar operator in Europe. He was employed with the Federal Aviation Administration for 31 years, retiring in 1973 as a control tower operator.

He founded Mercy Flights Inc., the nation's only non-profit air ambulance service, in 1949 and served as its chairman and chief pilot. Later he founded ACORDE Inc., an organization concerned with the rights of pilots.

In 1976 he was elected Oregon Pilot of the Year by the Oregon Pilots Association and in 1973 received the Oregon State Board of Aeronautics Award for outstanding service to aviation.

In addition to being a member of the Oregon Pilots Association, Mr. Milligan was a past president of the Rogue River Valley Knife and Fork Club, and a member of First Presbyterian Church, Medford.

Following his retirement he received a bachelor of law degree.

Survivors, in addition to his wife, include two sons, George Michael Milligan, Seattle, and Marc Prentice, West Linn, Ore.; two daughters, Ruth Ballweg, Seattle, and Virginia Olmscheid, Portland; his mother, Edna F. Milligan, Fair Oaks, Calif.; one brother, Richard J. Milligan, Fair Oaks, Calif., and seven grandchildren.

George Milligan's obituary in the *Medford Mail Tribune* detailed his career in aviation and his leadership in the community. The Nazarene Church, with the largest sanctuary in the area, volunteered their space for a crowded memorial service, which was followed by an open-invitation potluck in the Mercy Flights hangar.

Dr. Hank Boehnke, a beloved pediatrician in the community, had touched the lives of many through his advocacy for children and his concerns about health-care access. He developed protocols for Mercy Flights' neonatal transport program and trained flight nurses and paramedics to provide support for newborns. His memorial service was held at his home church, St. Mark's Episcopal Church, and was overflowing with close friends and grateful patients.

Pilot Bill Warren was a colorful figure. A respected pilot, he ran his own business as a crop duster, flew for Mercy Flights, and was an accomplished pilot in "The Great American Flying Circus," which raised money for Mercy Flights. Warren's moving tribute, "Message to George Milligan From Your Friends Back Here on Earth," was published and read at the memorial service after the February 1985 crash. (Courtesy of the Southern Oregon Historical Society.)

Boehnke service planned

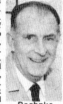

The memorial service for Dr. Henry L. Boehnke, 56, of Medford, who died Saturday, will be at 1 p.m. Wednesday in St. Mark's Episcopal Church, Medford, with the Revs. Warren P. Frank and Richard McDonald officiating. Perl Funeral Home is in charge of arrangements.

Boehnke

Memorial contributions may be made to Mercy Flights Inc., P.O. Box 522, Medford.

Dr. Boehnke was born July 21, 1928, in Eugene where he attended school. On July 1, 1951, in Eugene, he married the former Dorothy C. Thomas, who survives.

He served with the U.S. Army Medical Corps 1947-48 at Fort Sam Houston Hospital, San Antonio, Texas. He attended the University of Oregon and was graduated from its Medical School in June 1955. He completed his internship in 1956 and his residency in pediatrics in July 1958.

He was in private practice for seven years, then 21 years ago became associated with Medford Clinic.

In 1984 he received a Meritorious Achievement Award from the University of Oregon for 28 years of volunteer service as a professor of clinical pediatrics at UO.

Dr. Boehnke passed the American Board of Pediatrics in 1960 and was elected a fellow in the American Academy of Pediatrics in 1963.

His professional memberships included North Pacific and Oregon Pediatric societies, and American, Oregon, and Jackson County Medical associations.

He received his pilot's license in 1977, his commercial pilot's license in 1979, his instrument rating in 1980, and multi-engine rating in 1982. He had more than 1,100 hours of flying as a command pilot. For the past five years he was a volunteer pilot with Mercy Flights Inc., also serving on its board of directors and as a medical adviser.

He was a member of the University Club, Mount Ashland Racing Association, Medford YMCA, Aircraft Owners Association, and the Oregon Pilots Association.

Survivors, in addition to his wife, include one daughter, Joan M.B. Smith, Medford; two sons, John E. Boehnke, Medford, and Bill H. Boehnke, Pullman, Wash.; one brother, George T. Boehnke, Eugene; and two grandchildren.

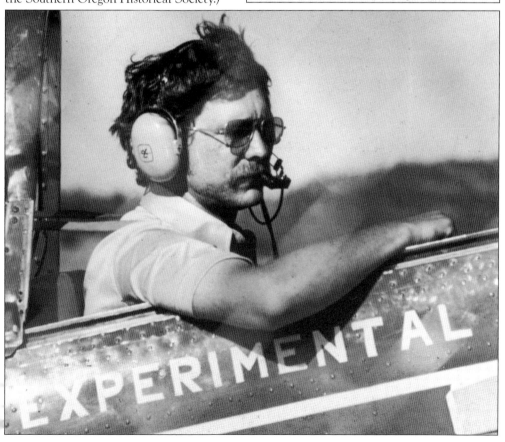

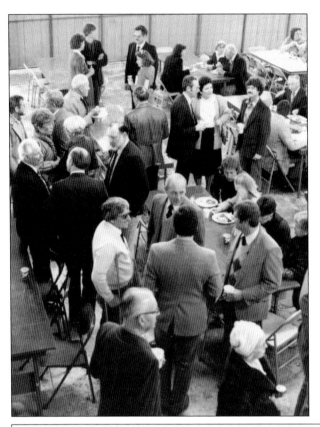

An open-invitation potluck at the Mercy Flights hangar followed Milligan's memorial service and was intended as a time for grieving, storytelling, and providing mutual support. The crowded hangar is pictured here filled with Mercy Flights family, friends, and community leaders in attendance. Longtime board member George Flanagan is at far left.

```
                                        2979 Barnett Rd., #203
                                        Medford, OR 97504
                                        Aug. 10, 1986

Dear Helene:

     I have had two great privileges in life. One is knowing and
loving George. The other is having some facility with words. It
was only natural that the two got together, and that they resulted
in a way to tell the world how so many of us feel about George
and the work he did, and how he did it.

     It is gracious of you to write as you did, Helene. If there
is nothing else, we'll always share the bond of our love for
George and all he stood for.

     There are still plenty of things wrong with my body, and I'm
in pain a good part of the time, but in the places where I feel
emotions and do my thinking I'm in pretty good shape.

     Thanks for your letter, Helene.

                                        Sincerely,

                                        Eric
```

Medford Mail Tribune editor Eric Allen, a close friend of George Milligan and longtime Mercy Flights board member and treasurer, wrote this letter of condolence to Milligan's wife, Helene.

Sen. Bob Packwood also wrote a condolence letter to Helene Milligan and the George Milligan family expressing thanks from him and his wife, Georgie Packwood, for George's "many years of service to the community and to Oregon."

BOB PACKWOOD
OREGON

United States Senate
WASHINGTON, D.C. 20510

February 13, 1985

Mrs. Helene Milligan
522 Mary Ann Drive
Jacksonville, Oregon 97530

Dear Helene:

Georgie and I just heard of George's passing. Words alone seem to be inadequate at a time like this. George contributed many years of service to the community and to Oregon. He will be sorely missed by all. Both Georgie and I want you to know that our thoughts are with you and the family.

Sincerely,

Bob

BOB PACKWOOD

BP/jt

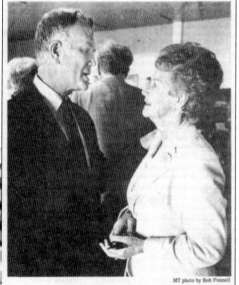

MT photo by Bob Pennell

Milligan honored

U.S. Sen. Bob Packwood chats with Helene Milligan at the Medford-Jackson County Airport after a ceremony Saturday to name the control tower for her late husband, George Milligan. Packwood introduced a bill to rename the tower shortly after Milligan died in a crash of a Mercy Flights air ambulance. President Ronald Reagan signed the bill Saturday. Milligan founded Mercy Flights, and once was a controller at the airport.

Sen. Bob Packwood is shown here with Helene Milligan at the celebration for the Medford–Jackson County Airport's renaming of the airport's control tower after George Milligan. The road leading to the Mercy Flights office and hangars was later named Milligan Way.

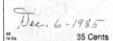

Dec. 6 - 1985

66
™ Co.

35 Cents

Mercy Flights says report was in error

By KAREN MERRILL
Mail Tribune Staff Writer

Mercy Flights directors say the National Transportation Safety Board erred when it challenged the competence of George Milligan, the pilot of an air ambulance that crashed Feb. 9 killing all four people aboard.

"In view of the evidence available, we find it difficult to believe and are suffering with indignation and dismay at the allegations made against our founder and friend, George Milligan," Mike Burrill, vice-chairman of the board of directors, said today.

"We do not know what happened that day nor what steps were used to initiate a recovery from a very serious situation that faced George. We do know that George was a very capable and competent pilot."

The NTSB this week issued a report blaming pilot error for the crash that killed Milligan, 65; Medford pediatrician Henry Lee Boehnke, 56; paramedic Steven Trosin, 39, and patient Marjorie Olney, 71, of Brookings.

The Mercy Flights air ambulance crashed and burst into flames about a mile short of a Medford-Jackson County Airport runway.

Burrill said Mercy Flights has requested, but has not yet received, a copy of the NTSB findings. Brad Dunbar, NTSB public information officer, has said the two-page report detailing the board's findings places most of the blame on Milligan.

"We determined there was no engine or fuel system malfunction," he said. "The board determined that the pilot lacked sufficient time and experience in this type of aircraft."

Burrill and Wayne Reavis, general manager of Mercy Flights, today passed out papers documenting Milligan's experience flying Aero Commanders, the type of plane involved in the crash. They said Mercy Flights has owned and operated five Aero Commanders throughout the years and at the time of the crash owned and operated two such aircraft.

Burrill said log book entries show that Milligan had logged more than 10,000 hours as pilot of an Aero Commander. He noted that the Federal Aviation Administration had certified Milligan as a trainer and tester of pilots who fly Aero Commanders.

Burrill said FAA inspectors tested Milligan in October and November of 1984 in the Aero Commander that was in the accident. The FAA tests include all normally anticipated emergency procedures, he said.

In its findings, the Transportation Board alleged Milligan did not know proper procedure for recovery from power loss, did not maintain sufficient speed in his descent, and improperly set the throttle for recovery from the power loss.

Burrill said the FAA certification checks Milligan passed in October and November included all normally anticipated emergency procedures.

"We feel our founder is being unfairly attacked," he said. "It almost appears to be a personal attack.

He added that the Mercy Flights directors will decide what action to take after they receive the NTSB findings. He said it's very likely they will appeal the decision.

Both Reavis and Burrill said they're concerned about the effect of the NTSB report on the reputation of Mercy Flights.

"If people think our chief pilot wasn't competent, what will they think about all of the pilots he trained?" said Burrill. "In my opinion, George was one of the best pilots around."

The cause of the February 9, 1985, crash remained controversial and raised questions about the FAA's investigation. The conflict received broad media coverage both regionally and nationally.

Wayne Reavis (left) and George Flanagan are pictured together with a Mercy Flights King Air. Reavis served in multiple roles including mechanic and manager. Flanagan was the original Mercy Flights treasurer for many years and used his business expertise to enhance the stability of Mercy Flights. Reavis and Flanagan played major roles in maintaining the stability of Mercy Flights after the 1985 crash. (Courtesy of the *Medford Mail Tribune*.)

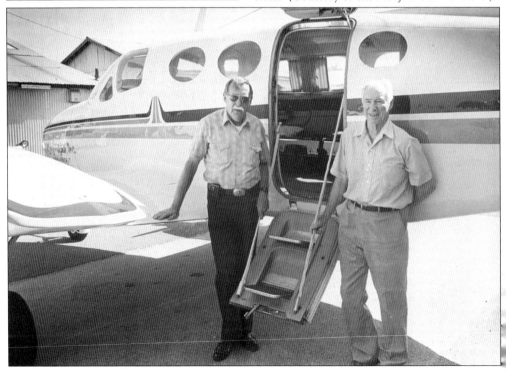

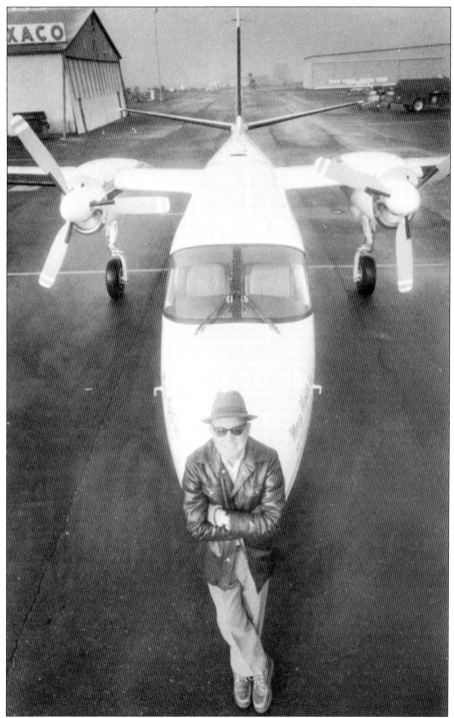

Posters using this image of George Milligan in front of an Aero Commander were displayed throughout the region to promote the 1985 airshow, which was dedicated to the memory of Milligan; proceeds from the show were donated to Mercy Flights. (Courtesy of the *Medford Mail Tribune*.)

Air ambulance crashes in Gold Beach

Plane hits power pole, killing crew of volunteers

The Associated Press

GOLD BEACH — A twin-engine air ambulance crashed Monday while trying to land at the Gold Beach airport, killing the three volunteer crew members on board.

Sheriff Chuck Denney of Curry County said the turboprop Beechcraft King-Air operated by Mercy Flights Inc. of Medford hit a power pole at 12:50 p.m.

Mercy Flights officials identified the dead as the pilot, Richard Mendolia, 40, of Medford; the co-pilot, Wally Nitowski, 48, of Eagle Point; and the flight nurse, Diane Lefler, 40, of Jacksonville.

The crash was the second in Mercy Flights' 40 years of volunteer service.

The plane was engulfed in flames as it tumbled into the front yard of a house at the end of the runway, Denney said.

The crash temporarily cut off power to part of this city of 1,585 on the southern Oregon coast.

Denney said the plane apparently strayed off course in fog as it made its approach to the airport.

The plane hit a parked truck and flipped over before coming to rest next to the house. The house and a boat were damaged by the heat from the flames.

There were no reports of anyone hurt or killed on the ground, Deputy Karen Baker said.

Federal Aviation Administration officials were heading to the scene to investigate, Baker said.

Mendolia and Nitowski were local commercial pilots, and Lefler worked at Ashland Community Hospital, Bob Cecil, the Mercy Flights operations director, said.

Mendolia was called in from the crew rotation list, and Nitowski and Lefler were already at Mercy Flights' office at the Medford-Jackson County Airport and volunteered to go when the call came in for a flight, Cecil said.

"They were here because they loved to be here," Cecil said with tears in his eyes. "It is love of man and love of flying that causes us to do what we do."

They were dispatched to pick up an 81-year-old woman who had suffered a stroke and bring her to Medford for treatment, Rex Strichler, the medical director for Mercy Flights, said. After the crash, the patient was taken by road to Medford.

The air ambulance service stopped operations for 24 hours to mourn the dead crew, Cecil said.

Mercy Flights was founded in 1949 to carry children suffering from polio from rural areas to hospitals in Portland.

In 1989, Mercy Flights lost its second aircraft. Pilot Richard Mendolia, copilot Wally Nitowski, and flight nurse Diane Lefler lost their lives in the small Oregon coastal town of Gold Beach as they were en route to pick up a patient being transferred back to Medford. This clipping from the *Statesman Journal* of Salem, Oregon, describes the crash and honors the dedication of the crew.

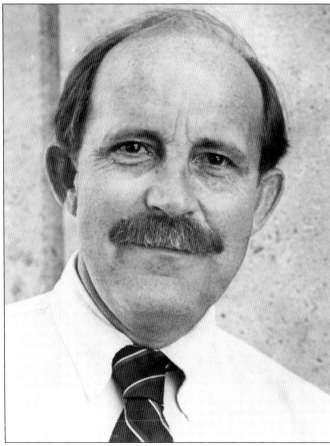

Bob Cecil was Mercy Flights' manager at the time of the 1989 Gold Beach crash. (Courtesy of the *Medford Mail Tribune*.)

Pilot Wally Nitowski is pictured at Mercy Flights headquarters at the Medford Airport. Nitowski was the copilot during the fatal crash at the Gold Beach airport in August 1989.

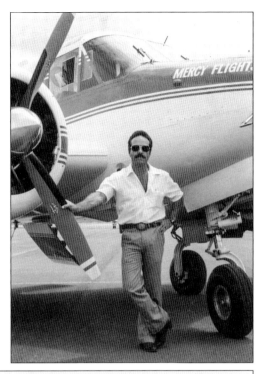

Mercy Flights crews, including pilots, paramedics, and nurses, continued to be committed to Mercy Flights' lifesaving missions. Pictured here are pilots Mike Newlun (left) and Jack Wheeler (center) and EMT Rick Yates.

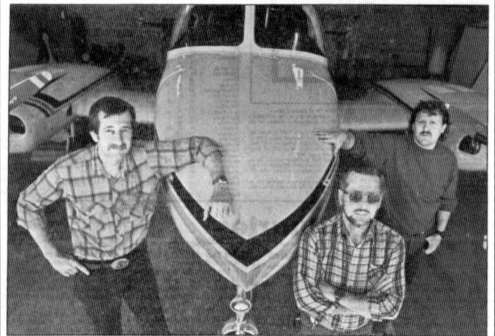

MT photo by Bob Pennell

Pilots Mike Newlun, left, and Jack Wheeler, center, and EMT Rick Yates are carrying on Mercy Flights tradition.

Mercy Flights carries on task

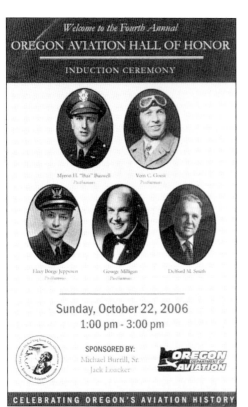

In 2006, George Milligan was posthumously inducted into the Oregon Aviation Hall of Honor at the Evergreen Aviation & Space Museum in McMinnville. The program for the event is shown here.

Pictured at the Oregon Aviation Hall of Honor induction ceremony in 2006 are George Milligan's daughter Virginia Olmscheid (third from left) and Michael E. Burrill Sr. (far left).

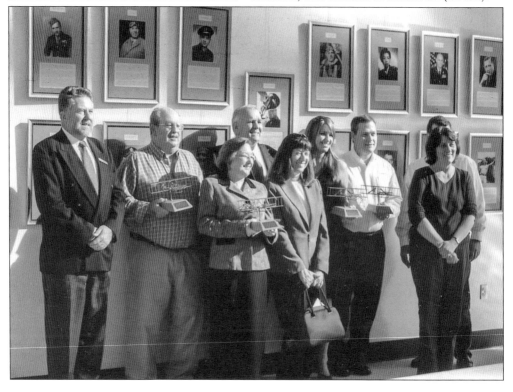

Seven

EXPANDING SERVICES

By the early 1990s, there were six ground ambulance companies serving the Rogue Valley. One of these providers, Medford Ambulance, was considering selling and had been approached by both of the hospitals in the area. The owner, Mike Hornbeck, made a decision that in hindsight seems very similar to the many decisions George Milligan made as he was forming Mercy Flights. Hornbeck did not want to see the hospitals control the ambulance services; he thought it would be in better hands with a community-owned organization like Mercy Flights.

Mercy Flights board chairman Jack James and Hornbeck got together and hammered out a deal for Mercy Flights to enter the ground ambulance business. Medford Ambulance provided the expertise and infrastructure, and Mercy Flights provided the long-term, community-owned leadership model, as well as an existing flight program. This decision was based on shared values between the two organizations, and many of the employees of Medford Ambulance were destined to become managers and executives of Mercy Flights in the future. It was a perfect match.

Within a few years, Mercy Flights had assumed responsibility for transport from three more ambulance companies, leaving three organizations providing service in the valley. Mercy Flights became the only community-owned ambulance provider in the Rogue Valley, and it was transporting more than 85 percent of the valley's patients.

The advantages of this business model immediately became clear. Decisions were made by a group of community members based on need and benefit to the community. Surpluses of the company could immediately be put toward new equipment and training. If it was good for the community, it was a priority for Mercy Flights.

In the years of the late-20th and early-21st century, it became obvious that the most effective way to bring critical patients from remote areas of the county to medical centers was via helicopter. In 1995, Mercy Flights started Southern Oregon's first air medical helicopter program. Mercy Flights made a deal to lease a helicopter and pilots from a local operator. They began flying Mercy Flights' nurses and paramedics to critical patients in remote areas. This was never a moneymaking venture for Mercy Flights, but it once again showed the versatility of a community-owned organization. If it was good for the community, the board and staff would find a way to make it work for the organization.

Conger-Morris Sells Ambulance Service

The sale of the Conger-Morris ambulance business, including one vehicle, records and good will, to Mr. and Mrs. Dayle Waltermire was announced Saturday by Carlos Morris, of Conger-Morris funeral home.

Conger-Morris began furnishing the ambulance service in 1945, and has continued to do so since that time.

Mr. and Mrs. Waltermire will use the business name, Medford Ambulance service, and have their business address at 30 Summit ave., but the ambulance itself will be garaged on West Main st., near Lincoln st. They will furnish 24-hour service, and Waltermire will devote full time to the business. He resigned as an employee of the California Oregon Power company yesterday. Mrs. Waltermire will stay on as a part time employee of Conger-Morris, where she has worked for some time.

Morris said any ambulance calls coming to his office will be relayed to the Waltermires. The new service's telephone number is 3-5001.

In the United States, ambulance service was also a component of the funeral home business. While it was not necessarily intentional, vehicles used by mortuaries to carry the deceased on stretchers were also the only vehicles large enough to transport the ill and injured. Shown here is a clipping from the June 13, 1954, issue of the *Medford Mail Tribune* marking the creation of Medford Ambulance as a spin-off of the Conger-Morris Funeral Home.

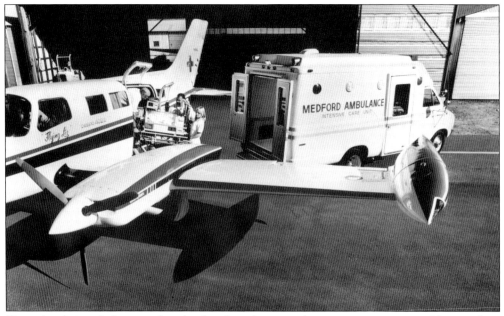

Ground and air ambulances go hand-in-hand, working together to transport patients. Here, workers with Medford Ambulance are transferring a neonatal patient to a Mercy Flights aircraft.

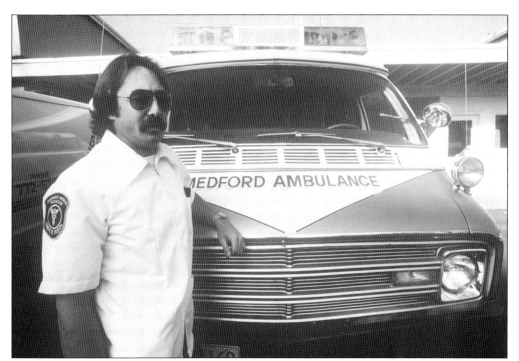

The merger between Medford Ambulance and Mercy Flights was instrumental in the history of both organizations. The common thread connecting them continues to be their management by a stable, community-owned organization.

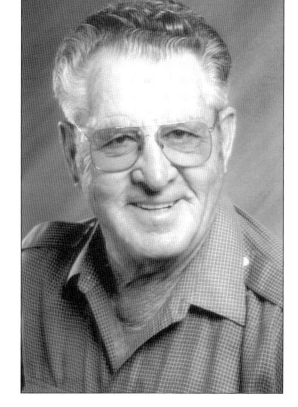

Medford businessman Jack James served on the Mercy Flights board as its chairman and was a key figure in building broad community support for Mercy Flights throughout local communities and service organizations. He worked with Mike Hornbeck of Medford Ambulance to bring the two organizations together.

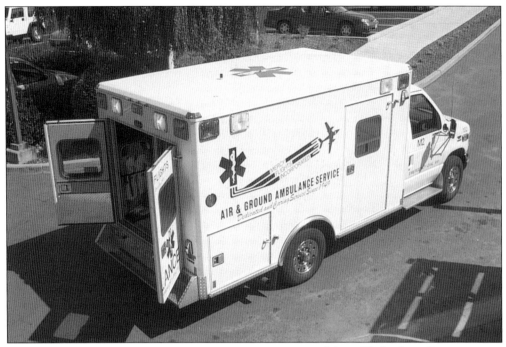

Mercy Flights branding was placed on the Medford Ambulance vehicles after the merger of the two organizations.

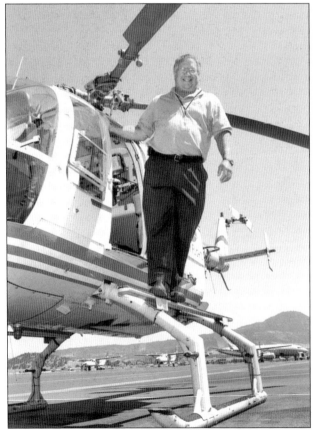

Ken Parsons started with Medford Ambulance in 1992 and moved over to Mercy Flights when the two organizations merged. He served in a variety of roles before being appointed CEO of Mercy Flights in 1996. (Courtesy of *Medford Mail Tribune*.)

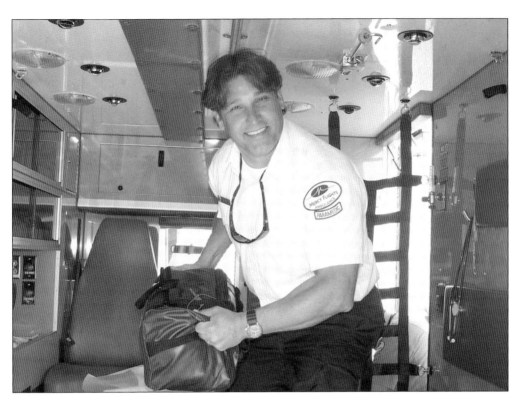

Doug Stewart started his career with Denver Health and Human Services in 1986 and worked there for eight years before relocating to Medford and joining Mercy Flights as a paramedic. He served in many roles during his 20-plus years with the organization before being appointed CEO in 2014.

Bob Ferreira, owner of Timberland Logging, saw firsthand the need for the medical transport of injured loggers, outdoorsmen, and others from remote areas throughout Southern Oregon. After adding a helicopter division to his business, he was unable to ignore the obvious connection of utilizing helicopters to move patients in the "golden hour"—the first hour following injury. He pushed his business partners to find a way to fill this need. (Courtesy of Tim Ferreira.)

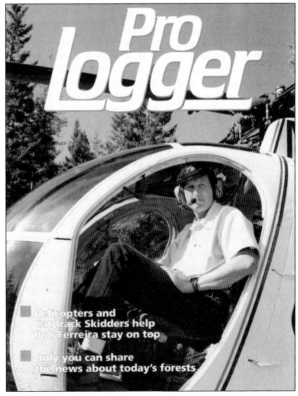

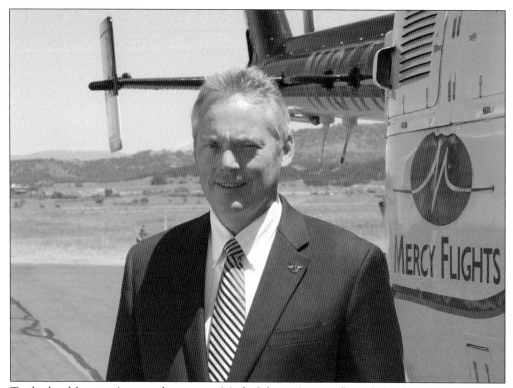

Timberland Logging's general manager, Mark Gibson (pictured), and chief pilot, Jeff Hubbell, were instrumental in the establishment of Southern Oregon's first air medical helicopter program in 1995. Charged by Bob Ferreira with making this a reality, they convinced the Mercy Flights board of the need for the service, negotiated a contract, and worked with the FAA and the Oregon Medical Board to obtain needed approvals to get the service up and running. For the first few years, Gibson and Hubbell carried radios with them 24-7 to monitor 911 calls and coordinate all details associated with getting a pilot, medic, and helicopter to those in need. (Courtesy of Mark Gibson.)

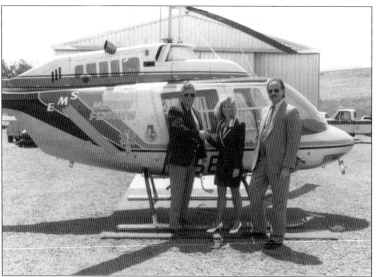

Ron Tycer (left) is shown with two unidentified hospital administrators as Mercy Flights began offering helicopter service, which included landing directly at hospitals as needed. The service—a joint operation between Timberland and Mercy Flights—utilized Timberland aircraft and pilots and Mercy Flights medical personnel.

Mercy Flights adds chopper service

By Pamela Lyons
Ashland Daily Tidings

4/11/95

The latest service offered by Mercy Flights will speed up medical care for victims of recreation accidents this summer.

Helicopter transport service began earlier this year as a third component in Mercy Flights' ambulance system. Helicopters provide faster transport to hospitals from remote areas where biking, rafting and skiing accidents are most likely to occur.

"This is going to be very lifesaving transports," said Pam Shrader, a paramedic for Mercy Flights. Shrader has flown on two of the six helicopter transports this year.

Mercy Flights, based in Medford, already provides ground transport service locally and air transport service to members throughout the West Coast with a twin-engine airplane.

The helicopter service is the first in Jackson County. The helicopters are flown by pilots for Timberland logging company, which works in cooperation with Mercy Flights for the program. Pilots remain on call for when emergencies arise and the helicopter launch pad on Dead Indian Memorial Road near Ashland.

Sunday, a motorcycle accident victim was transported from a remote area along the Rogue River to Rogue River Medical Center. It took the helicopter 36 minutes to make the flight.

copter has room for only one paramedic, who sits behind the pilot on a cushion about one-inch thick and has no back cushioning. The patient lies along the sides of the pilot and the

with their feet out a window, Shrader said.

Most patients are taken to Rogue Valley Medical Center or Providence Medical Center, Shrader

dents are common and the roads are often icy and dangerous.

"There's a lot of need for it because of uncertain conditions making ground transportation so

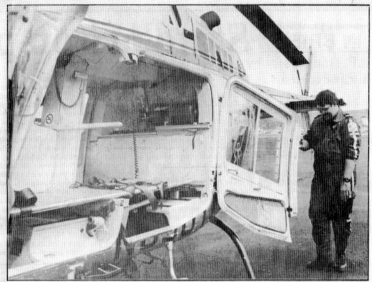

Ashland Daily Tidings/Pamela Lyons

Chuck Tiller, paramedic with Mercy Flights, shows the equipment inside the helicopter.

This article in the April 11, 1995, issue of the *Daily Tidings* highlights the new Mercy Flights helicopter service. This photograph of the first helicopter shows there was only room on board for three people: the pilot, patient, and medic. With the stretcher positioned so that the patient's feet were next to the pilot, the medic had access to the patient's upper body to provide critical care while airborne if needed. (Courtesy of the *Ashland Daily Tidings*.)

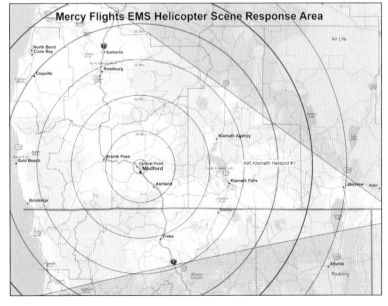

Helicopter service is available within a 150-mile radius of Medford, Oregon. This map helped emergency dispatchers visualize the response area. (Courtesy of H. Dashper Wood III.)

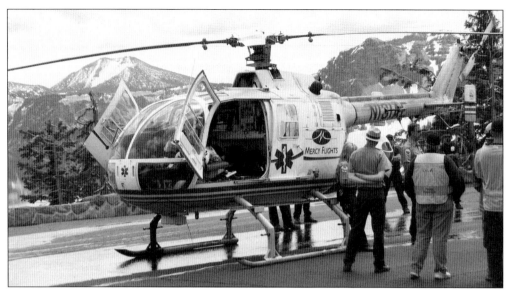

Training was critical to the successful rollout of the Mercy Flights helicopter service. They held sessions with emergency medical personnel in remote locations so people would be prepared for helicopter evacuations if needed. Here, the helicopter team is shown working with rangers and staff at Crater Lake National Park. (Courtesy of H. Dashper Wood III.)

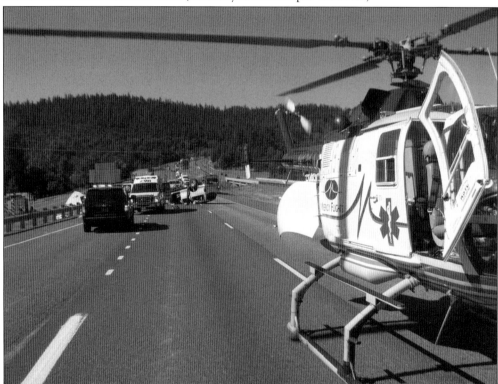

One of the benefits of helicopter rescue is the ability for helicopters to land directly at the scene of an accident or disaster. Here, Mercy Flights crew members are responding to an emergency call just outside of Grants Pass. (Courtesy of H. Dashper Wood III.)

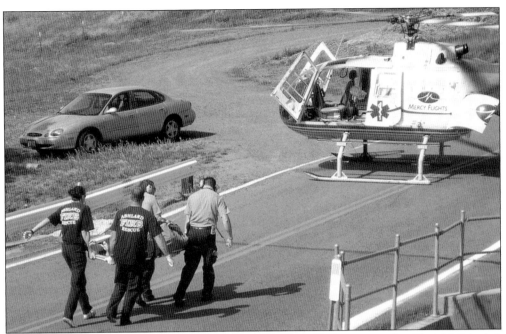

Pictured on the scene at Emigrant Lake in June 2008, Mercy Flights paramedics Chris Hall (at left in polo shirt) and Mike Ostrom (at right in polo shirt) work with two members of the Ashland Fire and Rescue team to load a patient for transfer. (Courtesy of H. Dashper Wood III.)

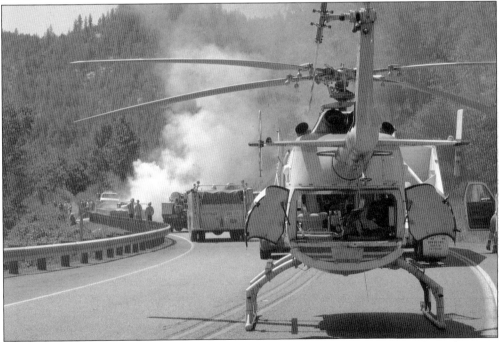

Like the early planes used by Mercy Flights, the first service helicopters needed to have doors cut into the aircraft to accommodate the loading and unloading of patients. Here, the FAA-approved doors are open awaiting patients from a multiple-vehicle crash on Highway 62 north of Shady Cove in August 2005. (Courtesy of H. Dashper Wood III.)

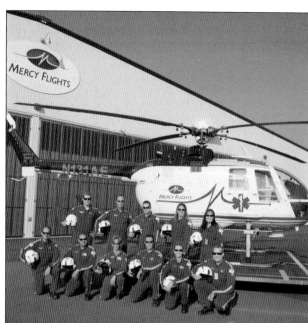

The 2012 helicopter and flight team is pictured in front of the new Mercy Flights hangar. (Photograph by Kai Cadarette; courtesy of H. Dashper Wood III.)

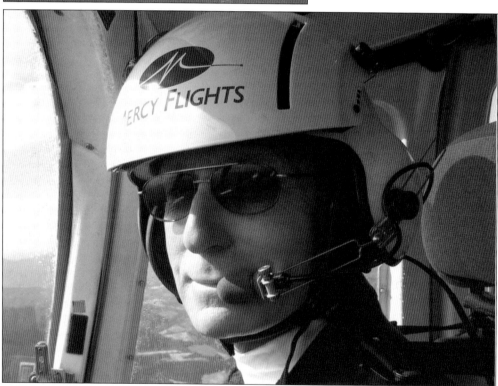

Timberland's chief pilot, H. Dashper Wood III, known as "Woody," flew with Mercy Flights from 2000 to 2015. After serving in the Vietnam War, he worked to gain experience flying a wide variety of aircraft as well as in pilot training and evaluation. This wealth of expertise made him well-suited to hire and train the right pilots for the Mercy Flights helicopter program. (Courtesy of H. Dashper Wood III.)

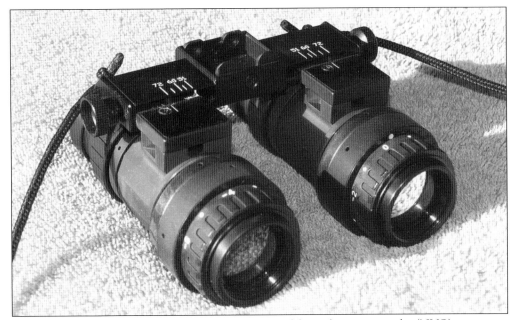

When Timberland and Mercy Flights received approval for night-vision goggles (NVG) operations by the FAA's Portland FSDO (Flight Standards District Office), it was the very first operation they had ever approved within the state. Although other EMS operations in Oregon were using NVG, they were supervised by FSDOs in other states such as Idaho, California, and Colorado. (Courtesy of H. Dashper Wood III.)

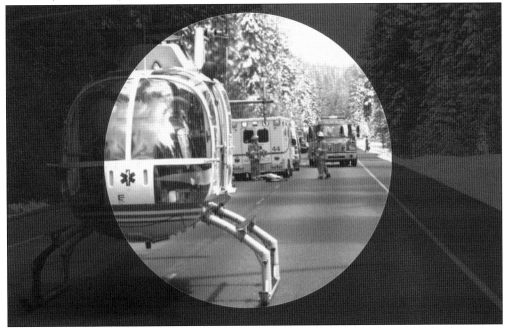

Heavily forested areas absorb ambient light, making night flights particularly challenging in Southern Oregon. Night-vision goggles enabled Mercy Flights to offer their helicopter service after sunset. As shown here, the goggles collect light that is invisible to the human eye and amplify it thousands of times. (Courtesy of H. Dashper Wood III.)

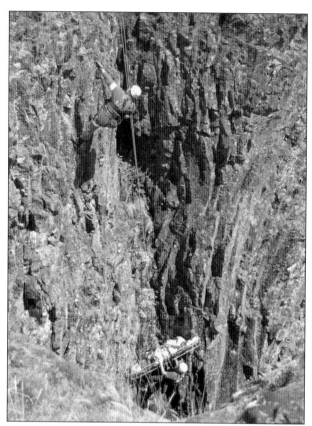

On May 21, 2006, while climbing a trail at Table Rock near Medford, a man decided to free climb a vertical wall above a crevasse. He fell and then slid another 30 feet into the crevasse. Pictured here are members of Fire District No. 3 guiding a Stokes basket containing the fallen man back up the face of the cliff. (Courtesy of H. Dashper Wood III.)

A Mercy Flights helicopter was used to quickly transport medical personnel and equipment from the staging area up to the rim. In addition to it being in a treacherous location, the rescue was complicated by a proliferation of poison oak and falling rocks. (Courtesy of H. Dashper Wood III.)

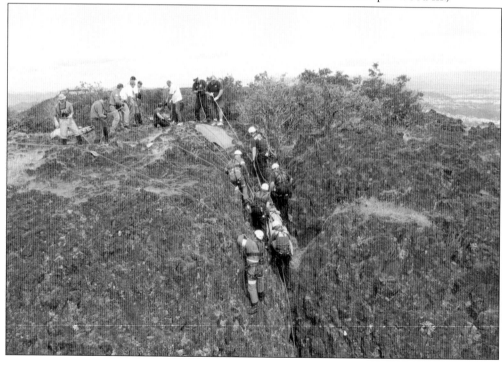

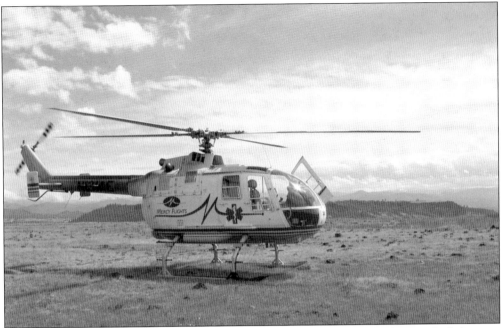

After the rescue, the patient was successfully transferred to a local medical center by helicopter for treatment. Mercy Flights and Jackson County's Fire District No. 3 were awarded unit citations for their teamwork and professionalism. (Courtesy of H. Dashper Wood III.)

Daring Rescue at Table Rock

Mercy Flights and Fire District #3 Receive Unit Citation from State

The State of Oregon recently honored Mercy Flights and Fire District #3 with the EMS Unit Citation, which recognizes exceptional emergency pre-hospital care and support activities under extreme circumstances.

Last Spring, a group was climbing off-trail at Table Rock near Medford. One man decided to free climb a vertical wall above a crevasse. After climbing approximately 50 feet, loose rock gave way and he fell. Upon hitting the ground, the man tumbled and slid down another 30 feet into the crevasse. His companions called 911 on their cell phone.

Mercy Flights and Fire District #3 quickly responded and set up a rescue staging area. Mercy Flights' helicopter was used to transport personnel and equipment from the staging area up to the rim to establish a rescue scene.

The rescue team quickly located the victim—he was in a dangerous spot where falling and tumbling rocks were a constant threat. To further complicate the situation, prolific poison oak growth covered the sides of the crevasse.

Rescuers lodged an all-terrain vehicle against a rock shelf with its winch. Three personnel were lowered into the crevasse with medical equipment and a Stokes basket. They treated the patient and carefully loaded him into the basket. At the top of the narrow crevasse, the team had to maneuver the basket from a horizontal to vertical position. The patient was successfully rescued and flown by Mercy Flights' helicopter to a nearby medical center for treatment.

For their teamwork and professionalism, Mercy Flights and Jackson County's Fire District #3 were awarded Unit Citations. Thank you to everyone involved for your individual and collective acts of heroism and perseverance. ∎

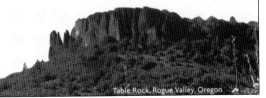

Table Rock, Rogue Valley, Oregon

This article in the Mercy Flights newsletter tells the story of the rescue at Table Rock.

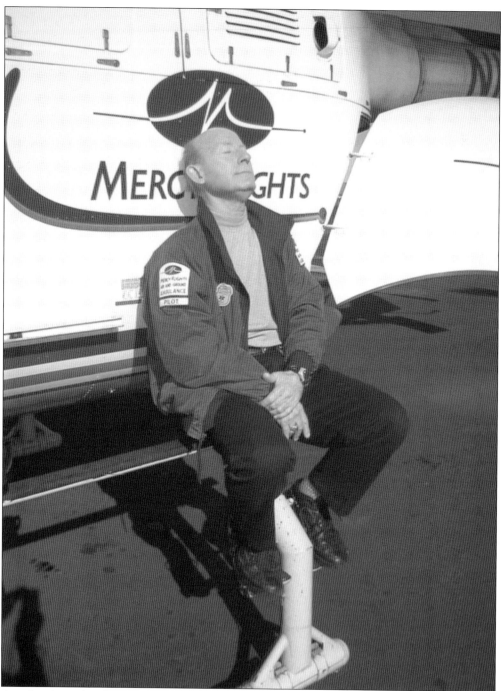

Another long day, but an optimal outcome! Timberland's chief pilot, H. Dashper Wood III (known as "Woody"), is shown catching his breath after a helicopter rescue. (Courtesy of H. Dashper Wood III.)

Eight

MOVING INTO THE FUTURE

Over the past three decades, Mercy Flights started making decisions its founders never would have imagined as helicopters, brand-new state-of-the-art maintenance centers and hangars, and modern training in technology and procedures in the nation's health-care system began a period of rapid change.

By 2006, Mercy Flights had purchased its second multi-engine turbine aircraft in response to increased demand for fixed-wing service throughout the region. The usage of its two Beechcraft King Airs, N117MF and N118MF, would continue to climb over the next decade.

By 2015, helicopter volume was consistently over 200 transports annually. Looking toward the future, the organization made a decision to purchase its first brand-new aircraft, a 2014 Bell 407GX helicopter. In keeping with tradition, the registration number was N119MF. With this purchase, Mercy Flights also began their own helicopter flight operation, becoming responsible for pilot training and all maintenance. This was a major step for Mercy Flights.

Mercy Flights is continuing to build infrastructure for the future. In 2011, the old hangars were torn down to make way for a new hangar and maintenance facility as well as additional offices and dispatch facilities. This $4-million expansion created a facility intended to serve the growing demand for air and ground services in the Rogue Valley.

Mercy Flights has experienced dramatic growth; by 2016, they were receiving more than 22,000 calls for service each year. Preparing the facilities and organization for the ever-changing future of health care is part of Mercy Flights' ongoing commitment to providing excellent service. Mercy Flights will always be on the forefront of technology and patient care. Providing caring customer service along with premium medical treatment and transport at a reasonable cost will always be the most important mission for Mercy Flights.

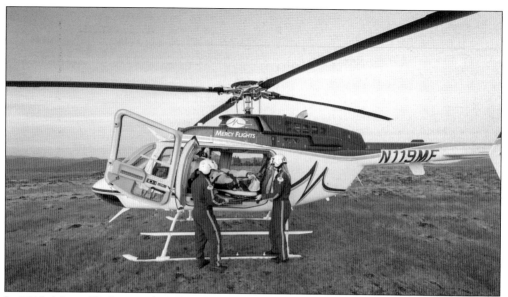

In 2015, Mercy Flights purchased its first brand-new aircraft, a 2014 Bell 407GX helicopter. With state-of-the-art electronics, it can fly far, fast, and with a high level of safety. Sticking with tradition, Mercy Flights gave the helicopter the registration number N119MF. (Photograph by Kai Cadarette.)

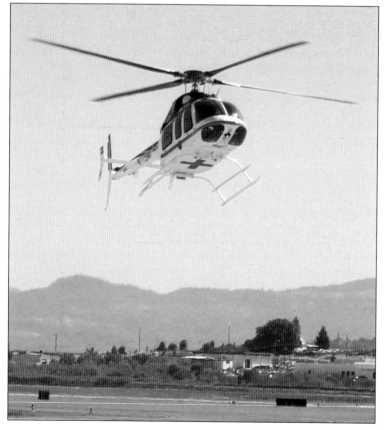

The bottom of the helicopter is marked with a red cross so that it can be easily identified as an emergency response aircraft upon approach.

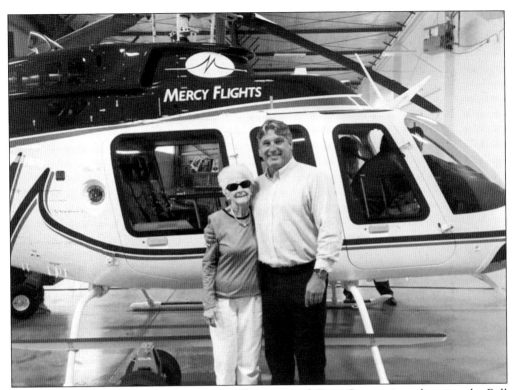

Helene Milligan (left), widow of George Milligan, joined Doug Stewart in welcoming the Bell 407GX to Mercy Flights' fleet.

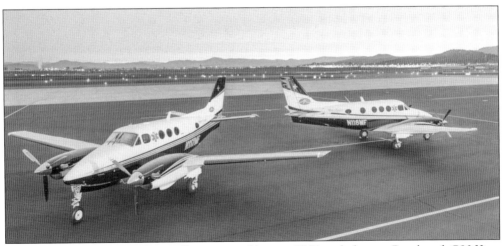

Mercy Flights' current fixed-wing fleet, pictured here in 2017, includes two Beechcraft C90 King Airs: N117MF and N118MF. (Photograph by Kai Cadarette.)

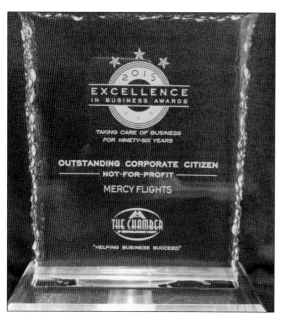

In September 2015, Mercy Flights was presented with the award of Outstanding Corporate Citizen (not-for-profit) by the Chamber of Medford/Jackson County.

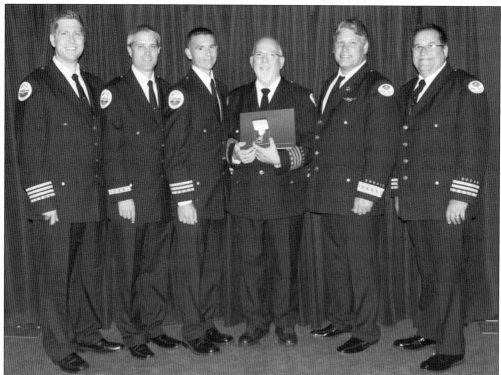

Mercy Flights paramedic Leslie Terrell (center) is pictured here after being awarded the EMS Cross Award at the Oregon State EMS Conference. The EMS Cross recognizes an EMT who, by act and deed, represents the most outstanding achievement in EMS over an extended period of time. This is the highest award that can be conferred in the absence of extreme conditions and extraordinary circumstances. Pictured with Terrell are members of the Mercy Flights team who were able to attend and show support for his outstanding achievement.

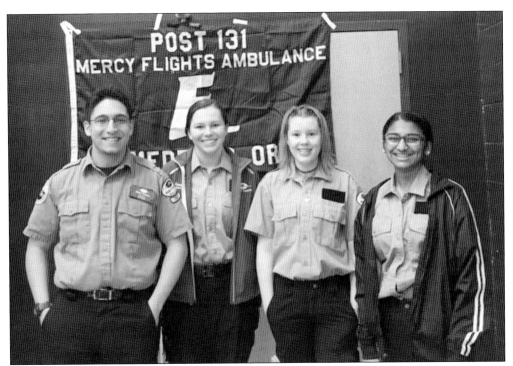

Through Explorers Post 131, Mercy Flights helps teenagers receive training and become Oregon Certified Emergency Medical Responders. Joining paramedics on ambulances in the Medford area, Explorers provide basic assistance to EMTs on emergency calls and educate and provide medical coverage at scout camps and other scouting events. Explorers also help to staff ambulances and first-aid stations at a variety of public and children's events. (Courtesy of Ed Sutton.)

Simulation training, with mannequins serving as patients, is used in medical education at all levels to teach medical procedures. In addition to benefitting the individual who is learning, simulation promotes team interaction in disaster and trauma management. Shown here is the Mercy Flights simulation room, which is used by paramedics to maintain and update their skills.

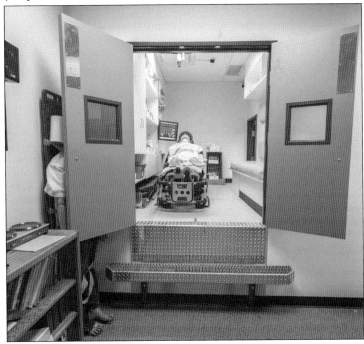

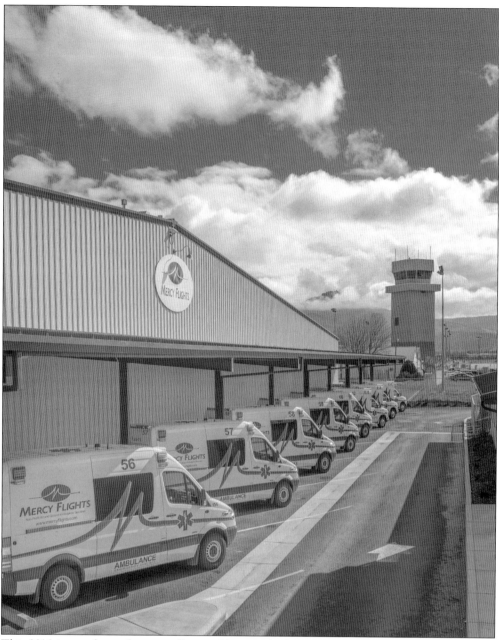

This 2016 image shows the new office and hangar facilities, as well as the new Mercedes-Benz Sprinter ambulances, which are economical in terms of fuel and maintenance. Mercy Flights plans to have their entire fleet converted to the Sprinter series by 2018. (Photograph by Kai Cadarette.)

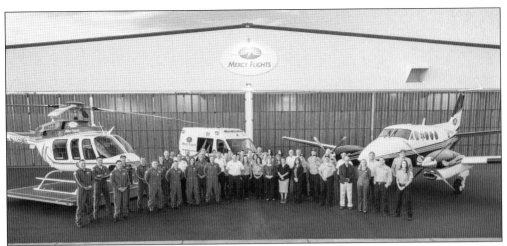

In addition to providing lifesaving services to the community, Mercy Flights has also become a valuable employer in Medford. By 2017, the number of paramedics, pilots, nurses, mechanics, and support staff employed by Mercy Flights had grown to a total of 126. (Photograph by Kai Cadarette.)

The 2017 executive team has a combined 50 years of service with Mercy Flights. Doug Stewart (left) was appointed chief executive officer in 2014 after working as a paramedic, field supervisor, director of medical operations, and the chief operations officer. Amy Hall (center) worked in multiple roles in accounting before being appointed chief financial officer. Tim James (right) served as paramedic, field supervisor, and medical operations manager until he was promoted to chief operations officer. Stewart and James both maintain current paramedic licenses. (Photograph by Kai Cadarette.)

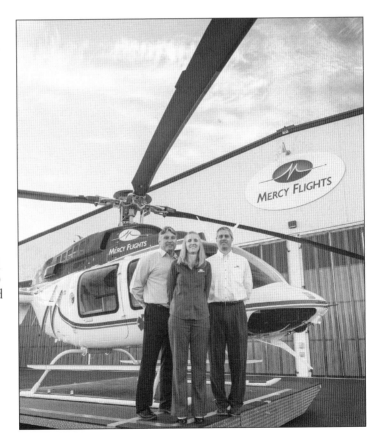

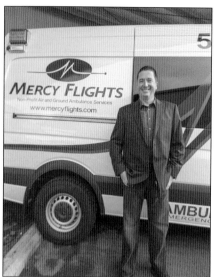

When Michael E. Burrill Sr. stepped down from the board of directors in 2008, his son Michael E. Burrill Jr. began his official service with Mercy Flights. "Mike Jr." went from member to treasurer to board chair (in 2013)—a position he still held in 2017 at the time this book was published. A respected local businessman and community leader, Michael E. Burrill Jr. also brings his experience as a commercial instrument–rated pilot to the organization. (Photograph by Kai Cadarette.)

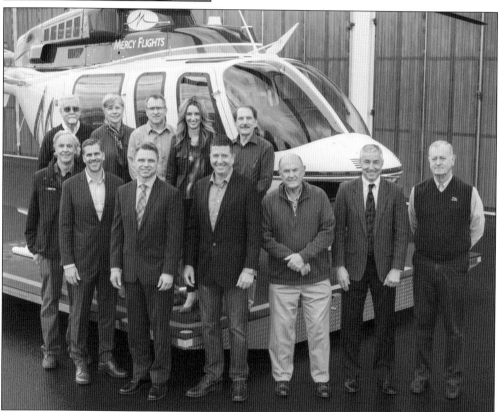

Continuing the tradition of a strong community-led board of directors, the 2017 board of Mercy Flights is shown standing in front of the organization's new helicopter. Pictured from left to right are (first row) Lou Budge, Mark DiRienzo, Greg Yechout, Michael E. Burrill Jr., Bruce Kellington, Richard Brewster, and Dale Gooding; (second row) Mark McQueen, April Sevcik, Mike Rudisile, Pirkko Terao, and Dr. Ed Helman. Not pictured are Heather Mackey, Brian McLemore, and board emeritus members Samuel James and Michael E. Burrill Sr. (Photograph by Kai Cadarette.)

BIBLIOGRAPHY

Atwood, Kay. *An Honorable History*. Medford, OR: Jackson County Medical Society, 1985.

Atwood, Kay, and Marjorie Lutz O'Harra. *Medford 1885–1985*. Medford, OR: Medford Centennial Committee.

Cole, Martin. *Their Eyes on the Skies*. Glendale, CA: Aviation Book Company, 1979.

Friedman, Ralph. *Tales Out of Oregon*. Sausalito, CA: Comstock Editions, 1972.

"Mercy Flights—a one picture story." *Ford Times* 47 (June 1955).

Milligan, George. *We Fly the White Birds*. Mercy Flights, 1983.

Morgan, Murray. "Oregon's Wings of Mercy." *Coronet Magazine* (June 1956): 82–84.

DISCOVER THOUSANDS OF LOCAL HISTORY BOOKS FEATURING MILLIONS OF VINTAGE IMAGES

Arcadia Publishing, the leading local history publisher in the United States, is committed to making history accessible and meaningful through publishing books that celebrate and preserve the heritage of America's people and places.

Find more books like this at
www.arcadiapublishing.com

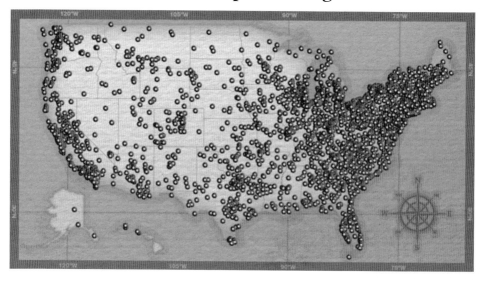

Search for your hometown history, your old stomping grounds, and even your favorite sports team.

Consistent with our mission to preserve history on a local level, this book was printed in South Carolina on American-made paper and manufactured entirely in the United States. Products carrying the accredited Forest Stewardship Council (FSC) label are printed on 100 percent FSC-certified paper.

MADE IN THE

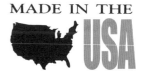